Intuitive Eating

OTHER BOOKS BY EVELYN TRIBOLE

Healthy Homestyle Cooking
(Rodale Books, 1994)

Eating on the Run
(Leisure Press, 1992)

Intuitive
EATING

....

A Recovery Book for the Chronic Dieter

Rediscover the Pleasures of Eating

and Rebuild Your Body Image

....

Evelyn Tribole, M.S., R.D., and
Elyse Resch, M.S., R.D.

St. Martin's Press ❧ *New York*

In the writing of this book, we have changed the names and occupations of all of our personal clients so that their true identities will not, in any way, be revealed, in order to maintain their anonymity. In addition, we use the pronouns *we* and *us* when referring to our work with individual clients, rather than specifying each time which of us has worked with a particular client. It should be noted, however, that each of us has a private clientele; we do not see clients together as a team. When referring to an event in the private life of either of us, we do differentiate between us by putting in parentheses the initials of the one involved—hence, (ET) refers to Evelyn Tribole and (ER) refers to Elyse Resch.

Design by Liney Li

Library of Congress Cataloging-in-Publication Data

Tribole, Evelyn.
    Intuitive eating : A recovery book for the chronic dieter/
Rediscover the pleasures of eating and rebuild your body
image/ Evelyn Tribole and Elyse Resch.
      p.   cm.
   ISBN 0-312-13097-X
   1. Reducing. 2. Nutrition. 3. Appetite. I. Resch, Elyse.
II. Title.
RM222.2.T717   1995
613.2'5—dc20   95-4018
                                        CIP

First Edition: May 1995

10 9 8 7 6 5 4 3 2 1

*To all of our clients and patients,
who have taught us so much.*

Acknowledgments

There are many people whom we would like to thank, without whose help, encouragement, and inspiration this book would not have been possible:

Arthur Resnikoff, Ph.D., for his feedback on the psychological principles used in this book.

Desy Safán Gerard, Ph.D., for her psychological support.

Sue Luke, R.D., and Elaine Roberts for their review and comments.

David Smith, our agent, who was instrumental in generating overwhelming interest in this concept.

Jennifer Weis, our editor, for her enthusiasm and support of Intuitive Eating and for her practical vision and input.

Tina Lee, editorial assistant, who cheerfully kept us on the straight and narrow with details.

Andréa Volz, secretarial assistant, for her endless hours in the library.

And lastly, our families and friends, whose unselfish understanding gave us the freedom to complete this book.

Contents

Foreword xiii

1. *Hitting Diet Bottom 1*

2. *What Kind of Eater Are You? 8*

3. *Principles of Intuitive Eating: Overview 20*

4. *Awakening the Intuitive Eater: Stages 31*

5. *Principle 1: Reject the Diet Mentality 41*

6. *Principle 2: Honor Your Hunger 61*

7. *Principle 3: Make Peace with Food 76*

8. *Principle 4: Challenge the Food Police 94*

9. *Principle 5: Feel Your Fullness 123*

10. *Principle 6: Discover the Satisfaction Factor 134*

11. *Principle 7: Cope with Your Emotions Without Using Food 147*

12. *Principle 8: Respect Your Body 164*

13. *Principle 9: Exercise—Feel the Difference 181*

14. *Principle 10: Honor Your Health—Gentle Nutrition 193*

Epilogue 213

Appendix: Common Questions and Answers About Intuitive Eating 216

References 221

Index 229

Foreword

If you could cash in every diet like a frequent flier program, most of us would have earned a trip to the moon and back. The $30 billion a year weight-loss industry could finance the trip for generations to come. Ironically, we seem to have more respect for our cars than for ourselves. If you took your car to an auto mechanic for regular tune-ups, and after time and money spent the car didn't work, you wouldn't blame yourself. Yet, in spite of the fact that 90 to 95 percent of all diets fail—you tend to blame yourself, not the diet! Isn't it ironic that with a massive failure rate for dieting—we don't blame the *process of dieting*?

Initially, when we ventured into the world of private practice we did not know each other. Yet separately, each of us had remarkably similar counseling experiences that caused us to rethink how we work. This led to a considerable change in how we practice and years later was the impetus for this book.

Although we practiced independently of each other, unknowingly each of us got started by making a vow to avoid the trap of working with weight control. We didn't want to deal with an issue that was only set up to fail. But while we tried to avoid weight-loss counseling, physicians kept referring their patients to us. Typically, their blood pressure or cholesterol was high. Whatever their medical problems, weight loss was the key to treatment. Because we wanted to help these patients, we embarked on the weight-loss issue with a commitment to do it differently: Our patients would succeed. They would be among that small 5 to 10 percent success group.

We created beautiful meal plans according to our patient's likes and dislikes, lifestyles, and specific needs. These plans were based on the widely accepted "exchange system" commonly used for diabetic meal planning and weight control. We told them that this was not a diet, for even back then we knew diets didn't work. We rationalized that these meal plans were not diets, because patients could choose among chicken, turkey, fish, or lean meat. They could have a bagel, a muffin, or toast. If they really wanted a cookie, they could have one (not five!). They could fill up with "free foods" galore, so that they never had to feel hungry. We told them that if they had a craving for a particular food, they could go ahead and eat it without guilt. But we also reinforced gently, yet firmly, that sticking to their personalized plan would help them achieve their goals. As the weeks went by, our clients were eager to please us, followed their meal plans, and, finally, their weight goals were met.

Unfortunately, however, some time later we started getting calls from some of these same people telling us how much they needed us again. Somehow, the weight had come back on again! Their calls were very apologetic. Somehow, they couldn't stick to the plan anymore. Maybe they needed someone to monitor them. Maybe they didn't have enough self-control. Maybe they just weren't any good at this, and definitely, they felt guilty and demoralized.

In spite of the "failure," our patients put all the blame on themselves. After all, they trusted us—we were the great nutritionists who had helped them lose weight. Therefore, *they* had done something wrong, not us. As time went on, it became clear that something was wrong with this approach. All of our good intentions were only reinforcing some very negative, self-effacing notions that our patients had about themselves—that they didn't have self-control, they couldn't do it, therefore they were bad or wrong. This led to guilt, guilt, guilt.

By this time, we had both reached a turning point in the way we counseled. How could we ethically go on teaching people things that seemed logical and nutritionally sound, yet triggered such emotional upheaval? Yet, on the other hand, how could we neglect an area of treatment that could have such a profound effect on a patient's future health?

As we struggled with these issues, we began to explore some of the popular literature that suggested a 180-degree departure from dieting. It proposed a way of eating that allowed for any and all food choices, without regard for nutrition. Our initial reactions were highly skeptical, if not downright rejecting. We reacted with self-righteous indignation. How could we, as nutritionists (registered dietitians), trained to look at the connections between nutrition and health, sanction a way of eating that seemed to reject the very foundation of our knowledge and philosophy?

The struggle continued. The healthy meal plans were not helping people maintain permanent weight control, yet the "throw-out nutrition approach" was a dangerous option. The suggestion to ignore nutrition and disregard how the body feels in response to eating "whatever you want" discounts the respect for one's body that comes along with the gift of life.

Eventually, we resolved the conflict by developing the Intuitive Eating process. This book is a bridge between the growing anti-diet movement and the health community. While the antidieting movement shuns dieting and hails body acceptance (thankfully), it often fails to address the health risks of obesity and eating. How do you reconcile forbidden food issues and still eat healthfully while not dieting? We will tell you how in this book.

If you are like most of our clients, you are weary of dieting and yet terrified of eating. Most of our clients are uncomfortable in their bodies—but don't know how to change. Intuitive Eating provides a new way of eating that is ultimately struggle-free and healthy for your mind and body. It is a process that unleashes the shackles of dieting (which can only lead to deprivation, rebellion, and rebound weight gain). It means getting back to your roots—trusting your body and its signals. Intuitive Eating will not only change your relationship with food, it may change your life.

We hope you find that Intuitive Eating will make a difference in your life, regardless of your weight goals—it has for our clients. In fact, when our clients learned that we were writing this book, they wanted to share some specific thoughts or turning points with you:

- "Be sure to tell them that if they have a binge, it can actually turn out to be a great experience, because they'll learn so much about their thoughts and feelings as a result of the binge."

- "Tell them that taking a time-out to see if they're hungry doesn't mean that they can't eat if they find they're not hungry. It's just a time-out to make sure that they're not eating on auto pilot. If they want to eat anyway, they can!"

- "When I come to a session, I feel as if I'm going to the priest for confession. That comes from all the times I used to go to the diet doctor, and I would have to tell him how I had sinned after he had weighed me. This isn't coming from you, but the inner Food Police."

- "I feel like I'm out of prison. I'm free and not thinking about food all the time anymore."

- "Sometimes I get angry, because food has lost its magic. Nothing tastes quite as good as it did when it was forbidden. I kept looking for the old thrill that food used to give me until I realized that my excitement in life wasn't going to come from my eating anymore."

- "With permission, comes choice. And making choices based on what I want and not on what somebody else is telling me, feels so empowering."

- "After giving up bingeing, I ended up feeling pretty low some of the time and even rageful at other times. I realized that the food was covering up my bad feelings. But it was also covering up my good feelings. I'd rather feel good and bad rather than not feeling at all!"

- "When I saw how much I was using dieting and eating to cope with life, I realized that I had to change some of the stress in my life if I ever wanted to let go of food as a coping mechanism."

- "Sometimes I have hungry days, and sometimes I have full days. It's so nice to eat more sometimes and not feel guilty that I'm going against some plan."

- "I get so exhilarated when I see a food I used to restrict. Now I think—it's free, it's there, and it's mine!"

- "I'm so glad you're writing this book; it will help me explain what I'm doing. All I know is that it works!"

- "When I'm in the diet mentality, I can't think about the real problems in my life."

- "This is the best I've ever taken care of myself in my life."

Chapter One

Hitting Diet Bottom

"I just can't go on another diet; you're my last resort." Sandra had been dieting all her life and knew she could no longer endure another diet. She'd been on them all—Slim-Fast, Jenny Craig, Scarsdale, Optifast, the grapefruit diet . . . diets too numerous to itemize. Sandra was a dieting pro. At first, dieting was fun, even exhilarating. "I always thought, this diet will be different, *this time.*" And so the cycle would recharge with each new diet, and every summer. But the weight lost would eventually rebound like an unwanted tax bill.

Sandra had hit diet bottom. By now, however, she was more obsessed with food and her body than ever. She felt silly. "I should have had this dealt with and controlled long ago." What she didn't realize was that it was the *process* of dieting that had done this to her. *Dieting* had made her more preoccupied with food. *Dieting* had made food the enemy. *Dieting* had made her feel guilty when she wasn't eating diet-type foods (even when she wasn't officially dieting). *Dieting* had slowed her metabolism.

It took years for Sandra to truly know that dieting doesn't work (yes, she was familiar with the emerging concept that dieting doesn't work, but she always thought she would be different). While most experts and consumers accept the premise that fad diets don't work, it's tough for a nation of people obsessed with their bodies to believe that even "sensible dieting" is futile. Sandra had been hooked into modern-age social mythology, the "big diet hope," for most of her life, since her first diet at the age of fourteen.

By the age of thirty, Sandra felt stuck—she still wanted to lose weight and was uncomfortable in her body. While Sandra couldn't bear the thought of another diet, she didn't realize that most of her food issues were actually *caused* by her dieting. Sandra was also frustrated and angry—"I know everything about diets." Indeed, she could recite calories and fat grams like a walking nutritional database. That's the big caveat, losing weight and keeping it off is not usually a knowledge issue. If all we needed to be lean was knowledge about food and nutrition, most Americans wouldn't have weight problems. The information is readily available. (Pick up any women's magazine, and you'll find diets and food comparisons galore.)

Also, the harder you try to diet, the harder you fall—it really hurts not to succeed if you did everything right. The best description for this effect is given by John Foreyt, Ph.D., a noted expert in dieting psychology. He likened it to a Chinese finger puzzle (a hollow cylinder of straw into each end of which you insert an index finger). The harder you try to get out, the more pressure you exert, the more difficult it is to get out of the puzzle. Instead, you find yourself locked in tighter . . . trapped . . . frustrated.

DIET BACKLASH

Diet backlash is the cumulative side effect of dieting; it can be short-term or chronic, depending how long a person has been dieting. It may be just one side effect, or several.

By the time Sandra came to the office, she had the classic symptoms of diet backlash. She was eating less food, yet had had trouble losing weight during her more recent diet attempts.

Other symptoms include:

• *The mere contemplation of going on a diet brings on urges and cravings* for "sinful" foods and "fatty favorites," such as ice cream, chocolate, cookies, and so forth.

• *Upon ending a diet, going on a food binge and feeling guilty.* One study indicates that postdieting binges occur in 49 percent of all people who end a diet.

• *Having little trust in self with food.* Understandably, every diet has taught you not to trust your body or the food you put it in. Even though it is the process of dieting that fails you, the failure continues to undermine your relationship with food.

- *Feeling that you don't deserve to eat* because you're over-weight.

- *Shortened dieting duration.* The lifespan of a diet gets shorter and shorter. (Is it no wonder that Ultra Slim-Fast's sales pitch is, "Give us a week . . . and we'll . . .")

- *The Last Supper.* Every diet is preceded by consuming foods you presume you won't eat again. Food consumption often goes up during this time. It may occur over one meal or over a couple of days. The Last Supper seems to be the final step before "dietary cleansing," almost a farewell-to-food-party. For one client, Marilyn, *every* meal felt like it was her last. She would eat each meal until she was uncomfortably stuffed—she was terrified she would never eat again. For good reason: She had been dieting over two-thirds of her life, since the sixth grade, through a series of fasting and 500-calorie diets. As far as her body was concerned, a diet was only around the corner—so she felt she had better eat while she could. Each meal for Marilyn was famine relief.

- *Social withdrawal.* Since it's hard to stay on a diet and go to a party or out to dinner, it becomes easier just to turn down social invitations. At first, social food avoidance may seem like the wise thing to do for the good of the diet, but it escalates into a bigger problem. There's often a fear of being able to stay in control. It's not uncommon for this experience to be reinforced by "saving up the calories or fat grams for the party," which usually means eating very little. But by the time the dieter arrives at a party, ravenous hunger dominates and eating feels very out of control.

- *Sluggish metabolism.* Each diet teaches the body to adapt better for the next self-imposed famine (another diet). Metabolism slows as the body efficiently utilizes each calorie as if it's the last. The more drastic the diet, the more it pushes the body into the calorie-pinching survival mode. Fueling metabolism is like stoking a fire. Remove the wood and the fire diminishes. Similarly, to fuel our metabolism, we must eat a sufficient amount of calories, or our bodies will compensate and slow down.

- *Using caffeine to survive the day.* Coffee and diet drinks are often abused as management tools to feel energetic and filled up while being underfed.

- *Eating disorders.* Finally for some, repeated dieting is often the stepping-stone to an eating disorder, ranging from anorexia nervosa or bulimia to compulsive overeating.

Although Sandra felt she could never diet again, she still engaged in the Last Supper phenomenon. We regularly encounter this when we see someone for the first time. She literally ate greater quantities of food than usual, and consumed plenty of her favorite foods because she thought she would never see these foods again. It's as if she were getting ready for a long trip, and were packing extra clothes. Just the thought of working on her food issues put her into the prediet mentality, a common occurrence.

While Sandra was just beginning to understand the futility of dieting, her desire to be thin had not changed—clearly a dilemma. She held on to the allure of the noble American dream.

THE DIETING PARADOX

In our society the pursuit of thinness (whether for health or physique) has become the battle cry of seemingly every American. Eating a single morsel of any high-fat or non-nutritionally-redeeming food is punishable by a life sentence of "guilt" by association. You may be paroled, however, for "good behavior." Good behavior in our society means starting a new diet, or having good intentions to diet. And so begins the deprivation cycle of dieting—the battle of the bulge and the indulge. Rice cakes one week, Häagen-Dazs the next.

"I feel guilty just letting the grocery clerk see what I buy," lamented another client, describing a cart stocked with fruits, vegetables, whole grains, pasta, and a small pint of *real* ice cream. It's as if we live in a food police state run by the food mafia. And there always seems to be a dieting offer you can't refuse. Exaggeration? No. There's a good reason for this perception. A study published in the 1993 *Eating Disorders—The Journal of Treatment and Preven-*

tion found that between 1973 and 1991, commercials for dieting aids (diet food, reducing aids, and diet program foods) increased tremendously.

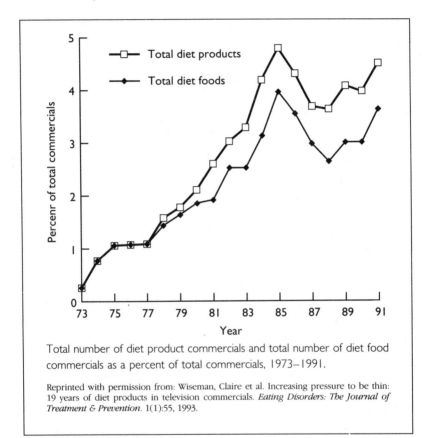

Total number of diet product commercials and total number of diet food commercials as a percent of total commercials, 1973–1991.

Reprinted with permission from: Wiseman, Claire et al. Increasing pressure to be thin: 19 years of diet products in television commercials. *Eating Disorders: The Journal of Treatment & Prevention.* 1(1):55, 1993.

The researchers also noted that there is a parallel trend in the occurrence of eating disorders. They speculate that the media pressure to diet (via commercials) is a major influence in the eating disorder trend.

The pressure to diet is fueled by more than television commercials. Magazine articles and movies contribute to the pressure to be slim. Even subtle cigarette billboards aim for the female Achilles heel, weight, with names such as Ultraslim 100, Virginia Slims, and so on. A new Kent cigarette, "Slim Lights," especially characterizes this focus on women's body issues. Their ad reads more like a commercial for a weight-loss center than for a cigarette by highlighting slender descriptions, "long," "lean," "light." Of course, the models in cigarette ads are especially slender. Lighting up as a weight-loss aid is not a new concept. As early as 1925, a Lucky Strike print ad campaign aimed at women stated, "To keep a slender figure . . . reach for a Lucky instead of a sweet." It is no surprise that the Center for Disease Control (CDC) attributed an increase in smoking by women to their desire to be thinner. Sadly, we have heard women in our offices contemplate taking up smoking again as a weight-loss aid.

But weight loss is not just a women's issue (although there's clearly added pressure on women). The proliferation of light beer commercials have planted the seed of body consciousness in men's minds as well—a lean belly is better than a beer belly. It's no coincidence that we've seen the launch of new magazines aimed at men, such as *Men's Fitness* and *Men's Health*.

While the pursuit of leanness has crossed the gender barrier, regrettably, we have given birth to the first generation of weight watchers. A disturbing new dieting trend is affecting the health of U.S. children. Shocking studies have demonstrated that school-age children are obsessing about their weight—a reflection of a nation overly concerned with diet and weight. Around the country, children as young as six years old are shedding pounds, afraid of being fat, and increasingly being treated for eating disorders that threaten their health and growth. Societal pressure to be thin has backfired on children.

Dieting not only does not work, it is at the root of many problems. While many may diet as an attempt to lose weight or for health reasons, the paradox is that it may cause more harm than good. Here's what our nation has to show for dieting:

- Obesity is higher than ever in adults and children.
- Eating disorders are on the rise.
- Childhood obesity has doubled over the last decade.
- There are more fat-free and diet foods than ever before, yet one out of three adults is overweight.

- Over 1,200 tons of fat have been liposuctioned from 1982 to 1992.

DIETING CAN'T FIGHT BIOLOGY

Dieting is a form of short-term starvation. Consequently, when you are given the first opportunity to *really* eat, eating is often experienced at such intensity that it feels uncontrollable, a desperate act. In the moment of biological hunger, all intentions to diet and desire to be thin are fleeting and paradoxically irrelevant. In those moments we become like the insatiable man-eating plant in the movie *The Little Shop of Horrors*, demanding to eat—"Feed me, feed me."

While intense eating may feel out of control, and unnatural, it is a normal response to starving and *dieting*. Yet so often, postdiet eating is viewed as having "no willpower," or a character defect. But when you interpret postdiet eating as such, it slowly erodes trust in yourself with food, diet after diet. Every diet violation, every eating situation that feels out of control, lays the foundation for the "diet mentality," brick by brick, and diet by diet. The seemingly brave solution—try harder next time—becomes as bewildering as the Chinese finger puzzle. You can't fight biology. When the body is starving, it needs to be nourished.

Yet so often a dieter laments, "If only I had the willpower." Clearly, this is not an issue of willpower, although glowing testimonials from weight-loss clinics often foster this incorrect notion. When underfed—whether from a self-imposed diet or starvation—you will obsess about food.

Maybe you don't diet, but eat vigilantly in the name of health and fitness. This seems to be the politically correct term for dieting in the nineties. But for many, it's the same food issue—with the same symptoms. Avoiding fat at all costs and subsisting on fat-free foods is essentially dieting, and often results in being underfed. There are many forms of dieting and many types of dieters. We will explore your dieting personality and meet the Intuitive Eater in the next chapter.

Chapter Two

What Kind of Eater Are You?

Perhaps you are still dieting and don't know it! There are many eating styles that are actually unconscious forms of dieting. Many of our patients have said they were *not* on a diet—but upon closer inspection of what and how they eat we found they were still dieting!

Here's a good example. Ted came in because he wanted to lose about fifteen pounds. He said that in his fifty years of living, he had only been on four serious diets. When perusing the book titles in the office (compulsive overeating texts, eating disorder books, and so forth) he stated, "You work with a lot of serious dieting problems . . . well I'm not one of those." Ted clearly did not see himself as a dieter, merely a careful eater. Yet it turned out that he was an unconscious dieter. Although Ted was not actively dieting, he was *undereating* to a level where he was nearly passing out in the afternoon. The reason—he had always been unhappy with his weight! In the mornings he would go for an intense hilly bike ride for one hour, then come home and eat a small breakfast. Lunch was usually salad with iced tea (while this sounds healthy, it's too low in carbohydrates). By suppertime, his body would be screaming for food. Ted was not only in a severe calorie deficit, but also carbohydrate-deprived. Evenings turned into a food fest! Ted had thought he had a "food volume" problem with a strong sweet tooth. In reality, he had an unconscious diet mentality that biologically triggered his night eating and sweet tooth.

Alicia also was not a conscious dieter. She came in not to lose weight, but because she wanted to increase her energy level. During the initial session, it became clear that she had complicated issues with food. So she was asked if she had been dieting a lot. She looked astonished. "How did you know that I've been on zillions of diets?"

While Alicia claimed to be okay with her current weight, she was still at war with food; she didn't trust herself with food. As it turns out, Alicia had been dieting since she was a child. Although she was not officially dieting, she retained (and expanded) a set of food rules with each diet that nearly paralyzed her ability to eat normally. We see this all the time, the hangover from dieting: Avoiding certain foods at all costs, feeling out of control the moment a "sinful" food is eaten, feeling guilty when self-imposed food rules are broken (such as "Thou shall not eat past 6:00 P.M."), and so on.

Unconscious dieting usually occurs in the form of meticulous eating habits. There can be a fine line between eating for health and dieting. Notice how even the frozen diet foods such as Lean Cuisine and Weight Watchers are putting their emphasis on health rather than diet. As long as you are engaged in some form of dieting, you won't be free from food and body worries. Whether you are a conscious or an unconscious dieter, the side effects are similar—the diet backlash effect. This is characterized by periods of careful eating, "blowing it," and paying penance with more dieting or extra-careful eating.

In this chapter, we will explore the various dieting/eating styles to help see where you are now. Later, you will meet the Intuitive Eater and the Intuitive Eating style, the solution to living without diets.

THE EATING PERSONALITIES

To help you clarify your eating (or dieting) style, we have identified the following key categories of eaters that exhibit characteristic eating patterns: the Careful Eater, the Professional Dieter, and the Unconscious Eater. These eating personalities are exhibited even when you are not officially dieting. It's possible to have more than one eating personality; although we find that there tends to be a dominant trait. Events in your life can also influence or shift your eating personality. For example, one client, a tax attorney, was normally a Careful Eater, but during tax season he became the Chaotic Unconscious Eater.

There's nothing wrong with possessing the eating characteristics described under the three eating personalities. But when your eating exists in one of these domains most of the time, it can be a problem.

Read through each eating personality and see which one best reflects your eating style. By understanding where you are now, it will be easier to learn how to become an Intuitive Eater. For example, you may find you have been engaged in a form of dieting, and not even have been aware of it. Or you may discover traits that unknowingly work against you.

The Careful Eater

Careful Eaters are those who tend to be vigilant about what foods they put into their bodies. Ted was an example of a Careful Eater (by day). On the surface, Careful Eaters appear to be "perfect" eaters. They are highly nutrition-conscious. Outwardly, they seem health- and fitness-oriented (noble traits admired and reinforced in our society).

Eating Style. There is a range of food behaviors that the Careful Eater exhibits. At one extreme, the Careful Eater may anguish over each morsel of food allowed into the body. Grocery shopping trips are spent scrutinizing food labels. Eating out often means interrogating the waiter—what's in the food, how the food is prepared—and getting assurances that the food is cooked specifically to the Careful Eater's liking (usually not one speck of oil or other fat used). What's wrong with this? Aren't label reading and assertive restaurant ordering in the health interest of most people? Of course! *The difference, however, is the intensity of the vigilance and the ability to let go of an "eating indiscretion."* Careful Eaters tend to undereat and to monitor the quantity of food eaten.

The Careful Eater can spend most of his or her waking hours planning out the next meal or snack, often worrying about what to eat. While the Careful Eater is not officially on a diet, his or her mind is—chastising every "unhealthy" or fatty food eaten. The Careful Eater can run the fine line between being genuinely interested in health, and eating carefully for the sake of body image.

Sometimes the Careful Eater is guided by time or events. For example, some Careful Eaters are meticulous during the weekdays, so that they earn their "eating right" to splurge on the weekends or at an upcoming party. But weekends occur 104 days of the year—

the splurges can backfire with unwanted weight gain. Consequently, it's not unusual for a Careful Eater to contemplate going on a diet.

The Problem. There's nothing wrong with being a Careful Eater and interested in the well-being of your body. The problem occurs, however, when diligent eating (almost bordering on militant) affects a healthy relationship with food—and negatively impacts your body. Careful Eaters, upon closer inspection, resemble a subtle dieting style. They may not diet, but they scrutinize every food situation.

The Professional Dieter

Professional Dieters are easier to identify; they are perpetually dieting. They have usually tried the latest commercial diet, diet book, or new weight-loss gimmick. Sometimes dieting takes place in the form of fasting, or "cutting back." Professional Dieters know a lot about portions of foods, calories, and "dieting tricks," yet the reason they are always on another diet is that the original one never worked. Today, the Professional Dieter is also well-versed in fat-gram counting.

Eating Style. Professional Dieters also have careful eating traits. The difference, however, is that chronic dieters make every eating choice for the sake of losing weight, not necessarily for health. When the dieter is not officially on a diet, he or she is usually thinking about the next diet that can be started. She often wakes up hoping this will be a good day—the new beginning.

While Professional Dieters have a lot of dieting knowledge, it doesn't serve them well. It's not unusual for them to binge or engage in Last Supper eating the moment a forbidden food is eaten. That's because chronic dieters truly believe they will not eat this food again; for tomorrow they diet, tomorrow they start over with a clean slate. Better eat now, it's the last chance. Not surprisingly, the Professional Dieter gets frustrated at the futility of the vicious cycle. Diet, lose weight, gain weight, binge intermittently, and go back to dieting.

The Problem. It's hard to live this way. Yo-yo dieting makes it increasingly difficult to lose weight, let alone eat healthfully. Chronic undereating usually results in overeating or periodic binges.

For some Professional Dieters, the frustration of losing weight becomes so intensified that they may try laxatives, diuretics, and diet pills. And because these "diet aids" do not work, they may try extreme methods such as chronic restricting, in the form of anorexia nervosa, or purging (throwing up after a binge), in the form of bulimia. While anorexia and bulimia are multifactorial and rooted with psychological issues, a growing body of research has demonstrated that chronic dieting is a common stepping-stone into an eating disorder. One study in particular found that by the time dieters reach the age of fifteen years, they are eight times as likely to suffer from an eating disorder as nondieters.

The Unconscious Eater

The Unconscious Eater is often engaged in paired eating—which is eating and doing another activity at the same time, such as watching television and eating, or reading and eating. Because of the subtleties, and lack of awareness, it can be difficult to identify this eating personality. There are many subtypes of Unconscious Eaters.

The Chaotic Unconscious Eater often lives an overscheduled life, too busy, too many things to do. The chaotic eating style is haphazard; whatever's available will be grabbed—vending machine fare, fast food, it'll all do. Nutrition and diet are often important to this person—just not at the *critical moment* of the chaos. Chaotic Eaters are often so busy putting out fires that they have difficulty identifying biological hunger until it's fiercely ravenous. Not surprisingly, the Chaotic Eater goes long periods of time without eating.

The Refuse-Not Unconscious Eater is vulnerable to the mere presence of food, regardless if he or she is hungry or full. Candy jars, food lying around at meetings, food sitting on a kitchen counter will not usually be passed up by the Refuse-Not Eater. Most of the time, however, Refuse-Not Eaters are not aware that they *are* eating, or how much they are eating. For example, the Refuse-Not Eater may pluck up a couple of candies on the way to the restroom without being aware of it. Social outings that revolve around food such as cocktail parties and holiday buffets are especially tough for the Refuse-Not Eater.

*The **Waste-Not Unconscious Eater*** values the food dollar. His or her eating drive is often influenced by getting as much as you can for the money. The Waste-Not Eater is especially inclined to clean the plate (and others as well). It's not unusual for a Waste-Not Eater to eat the leftovers from children or spouse.

*The **Emotional Unconscious Eater*** uses food to cope with emotions, especially uncomfortable emotions such as stress, anger, and loneliness. While Emotional Eaters view their eating as *the* problem, it's often a symptom of a deeper issue. Eating behaviors of the Emotional Eater can range from grabbing a candy bar in stressful times to chronic compulsive binges of vast quantities of food.

*The **Problem*.** Unconscious eating in its various forms is a problem if it results in chronic overeating (which can easily occur when you are eating and not quite aware of it).

Keep in mind that somewhere *between* the first and last bite of food is where the lapse of consciousness takes place. As in, "Oh, it's all gone!" For example, have you ever bought a large box of candy at the movies and begun to eat it only to discover your fingers *suddenly* scraping the bottom of the empty box? That's a simple form of unconscious eating. But unconscious eating can also exist at an intense level, in a somewhat altered state of eating. In this case, the person is not aware of what is being eaten, why he started eating, or even how the food tastes. It's like zoning out with food.

WHEN YOUR EATING PERSONALITY
WORKS AGAINST YOU

Eventually, the eating styles of the Careful Eater, the Professional Dieter, and the Unconscious Eater become an ineffective way of eating, even when on the surface they appear okay. The solution for the frustrated eater: Try harder with a new diet! At first the new diet seems exhilarating and hopeful, but eventually the familiar pounds return. Dieting gets more difficult, and even when you resume your baseline eating personality, it may feel more uncomfortable than before. This is because with each diet the inner food rules get stronger. These food rules often perpetuate feelings of guilt about eating even when you are not officially dieting. Also, the biological effects of dieting (as detailed in Chapter 5) make it increasingly difficult to have a normal relationship with food.

The Intuitive Eater personality, however, is the exception. It is the one eating style that doesn't work against you, and can help you end chronic dieting and yo-yo weight fluctuations.

INTRODUCING THE INTUITIVE EATER

Intuitive Eaters march to their inner hunger signals, and eat whatever they choose without experiencing guilt or an ethical dilemma. The Intuitive Eater is an unaffected eater. Yet it is increasingly difficult to be an unaffected eater in today's health-conscious society when you consider the bombardment of nutrition, food, and weight messages from commercials, media, and health professionals.

When we've described the basic eating traits of the Intuitive Eater to our clients, it's amazing how often we'll hear the response, "That's how my wife eats" or "That's how my boyfriend eats." When we ask how that person's weight and relationship to food are, the response is, "No problem!"

Consider toddlers. They are the natural Intuitive Eaters— virtually free from societal messages about food and body image. Toddlers have an innate wisdom about food if you don't interfere with it. They don't eat based on dieting rules or health, yet study after study shows that if you let a toddler eat spontaneously, he will eat what he needs when given free access to food. (This is probably the toughest thing for a concerned parent to do—to let go and trust that kids have an innate ability to eat!)

A landmark study led by Leann Birch, Ph.D., and published in the *New England Journal of Medicine* confirmed that preschool-aged children have an innate ability to regulate their eating according to what their bodies need for growth. This holds true even when, meal by meal, the little tykes' eating appears to be a parent's nightmare. Researchers found that at a given meal, calorie intake was highly variable, but it balanced out over time. Yet, many parents assume that their young children cannot adequately regulate their food intake. Consequently, parents often adopt coercive strategies in an attempt to ensure that the child consumes a nutritionally adequate diet. But previous research by Birch and her colleagues indicates that such *control* strategies are counterproductive.

Furthermore, Birch notes that *"parents' attempts to control their child's eating were reported more often by obese adults than by adults of normal weight."* Similarly, Duke University psychologist Philip Costanzo, Ph.D., found that excess weight in school-age children was highly associated with the degree to which parents tried to restrain their children's eating. Even well-meaning parents interfere with intuitive eating. When a parent tries to overrule a child's natural eating cues, the problem gets worse, not better.

A parent who feeds a child whenever a hunger signal is heard and who stops feeding when the child shows that he's had enough, can play a powerful role in the initial development of Intuitive Eating.

In fact, groundbreaking work by therapist and dietitian Ellyn Satter has shown that if you get the parents of overweight kids to back off, and let them eat without parental pressure, the kids will eventually eat *less*. Why? The child begins to hear and understand his own inner signals of hunger and satiety. The child also knows that he or she will have access to food.

According to Satter, "Children deprived of food in an attempt to be thin become preoccupied with food, afraid they won't get enough to eat, and are prone to overeat when they get the chance." We have found this to be true for adult dieters as well. Only for adults, the intuitive eating process has been buried for a long time, often years and years. Instead of having a parent loosen up the pressure, this loosening of pressure has to come from within. And against society's myth of dieting and distorted body worship.

Fortunately, *we all possess the natural intuitive eating ability*; it's just been suppressed, especially by dieting. This book is devoted to showing you how to awaken the Intuitive Eater within.

SUMMARY OF EATING STYLES

Eating Style	Trigger	Characteristic
Careful Eater	Fitness and health	Appears to be the perfect eater. Yet anguishes over each food morsel and its effect on the body. On the surface, this person seems health- and fitness-oriented.
Unconscious Eater	Eating while doing something else at the same time	This person is often unaware that she/he is eating, or how much is being eaten. To sit down and simply eat, is often viewed as a waste of time. Eating is usually paired with another activity to be productive. There are many subtypes.
Chaotic Unconscious Eater	Overscheduled life	This person's eating style is haphazard— gulp 'n go when the food is available. Seems to thrive on tension.
Refuse-Not Unconscious Eater	Presence of food	This person is especially vulnerable to candy jars, or food present in meetings or sitting openly on the kitchen counter.
Waste-Not Unconscious Eater	Free food	This person's eating drive is often influenced by the value of the food dollar and is susceptible to all-you-can-eat buffets and free food.

SUMMARY OF EATING STYLES (*cont.*)		
Eating Style	Trigger	Characteristic
Emotional Unconscious Eater	Uncomfortable emotions	Stress or uncomfortable feelings trigger eating—especially when alone.
Professional Dieter	Feeling fat	This person is perpetually dieting, often trying the latest commercial diet or diet book.
Intuitive Eater	Biological hunger	This person makes food choices without experiencing guilt or an ethical dilemma. Honors hunger, respects fullness, enjoys the pleasure of eating.

HOW YOUR INTUITIVE EATER GETS BURIED

As toddlers get a little older, mixed messages begin to creep in—from the early influences of the Saturday morning food commercial, to the well-meaning parent who coaxes, "Clean your plate." The assault does not stop when you are a child. There are several external forces that influence your eating, which can further bury intuitive eating.

Dieting. You have already seen the damage that chronic dieting plays, including but not limited to:

- Increased binge eating
- Decreased metabolic rate
- Increased preoccupation with food
- Increased feelings of deprivation

- Increased sense of failure
- Decreased sense of willpower

This only serves to erode your trust with food and urges you to rely on *external* sources to guide your eating (a food plan, a diet, the time of day, food rules, and so forth). The more you go to external sources to "judge" if your eating is in check, the *further* removed you become from Intuitive Eating. Intuitive Eating relies on *your own* internal cues and signals.

Eat-Healthfully-or-Die Messages. Messages about eating healthfully are everywhere, from nonprofit health organizations to food companies touting the health benefits of their particular product. The inherent message? What you eat can improve your health. Conversely, take one wrong move (bite) and you're one step closer to the grave. Is this an exaggeration? No. For example, a 1994 press release issued by the Harvard School of Public Health stated that eating trans fatty acids (found in margarine) may cause 30,000 deaths each year in the United States from heart disease. That kind of message can easily leave you feeling guilty for eating the "wrong" kind of food and confused about what you should eat.

Magazine and newspapers have also greatly increased their coverage of food and health. One food editor, Joe Crea, of a major metropolitan newspaper, the *Orange County Register* (California), noted that in a six-year period (1987–1993), his stories on nutrition increased fivefold. Of nearly eight hundred food stories, two hundred were on health-related issues. While there is no doubt that what you eat can have an impact on your health, the exponential increase in media coverage has served as a conduit to building food paranoia in the consumer, especially the dieter. Joe Crea agrees. "You open the paper, see a beautiful lead story about cheesecake, and simultaneously another piece on how overeating will make you fat. It puts the reader in conflict."

Are we saying that you should ignore the virtues of healthful eating? Of course not. However, when you have a dieting mind-set, the barrage of healthy-eating messages can make you feel guiltier about the food you choose to eat. *Obesity and Health* reported a survey on 2,075 adults in Florida that revealed that 45 percent of adults felt *guilty* after eating foods they like. (Keep in mind that this survey was conducted to reflect typical American demographics. These "guilt-by-eating" numbers would most likely be much higher if performed on dieters.)

Women may be especially guilt-ridden. An American Dietetic Association Gallup poll showed that women feel guiltier than men about the food they eat (44 percent versus 28 percent). Could this be because women diet more frequently than men? Or because women are usually the target of health messages and food ads (consider the number of women's magazines). Women are the key decision makers for the health care for the family, and are usually the gatekeepers of food and nutrition issues as well; they serve as a prime target.

We have found that establishing nutrition or healthy eating as an *initial* priority in the Intuitive Eating process is counterproductive. In the beginning we *ignore* nutrition, because it interferes with the process of re-learning how to become an Intuitive Eater. Nutrition heresy? No. It's possible to respect and honor nutrition. It just can't be the first priority when you've been dieting all your life. Or look at it this way, if you have focused all your attention on nutrition, has it helped? People can embrace even the most nutritious eating plan (including counting fat grams) as another form of diet.

You can recapture Intuitive Eating, but first you have to get rid of the diet mentality rules that keep the Intuitive Eater buried. In the next chapter, we will briefly introduce you to the core principles of Intuitive Eating. The remainder of the book will show you step by step how to become an Intuitive Eater.

....

Chapter Three

Principles of Intuitive Eating: Overview

Only when you vow to discard dieting and replace it with a commitment to Intuitive Eating will you be released from the prison of yo-yo weight fluctuations and food obsessions.

In this chapter, you will be introduced to the core principles of Intuitive Eating—just a snapshot essence of each concept, with a brief case study or two. While in many of these cases, our clients lost weight, the most significant achievement for them was gaining a healthy relationship with food and their bodies. By following the ten principles of Intuitive Eating, you will normalize your relationship with food. How this affects your weight depends on your existing eating style and attitude toward your body.

Later in the book, each principle will be discussed step by step in great detail. You may find it useful to return to this chapter for a quick reference.

PRINCIPLE 1:

REJECT THE DIET MENTALITY

Throw out the diet books and magazine articles that offer you the false hope of losing weight quickly, easily, and permanently. Get angry at the lies that have led you to feel as if you were a failure every time a new diet stopped working and you gained back all of the weight. If you allow even one small hope to linger that a new and better diet might be lurking around the corner, it will prevent you from being free to rediscover Intuitive Eating.

James dieted most of his life, starting with the little diets his mother put him on and ending with a liquid protein fast which gave him his most recent short-lived "success." By the time he came in, James weighed more than he ever had in his life. He knew he was incapable of ever going on another diet but felt guilty because he thought he "should." *Rejecting the diet mentality* was a key milestone for James. He discovered that he was not a failure, but that the system of dieting itself created the set-up for failure.

Today, James is a committed ex-dieter who found his way back through Intuitive Eating. He no longer feels that he "should" be on a diet. He is pleased and amazed that he has lost twenty-five pounds while eating everything he likes. Now, James sadly watches others go from diet to diet, while he himself realizes that dieting is the quickest short-circuit to a healthy relationship with food.

PRINCIPLE 2:

HONOR YOUR HUNGER

Keep your body fed biologically with adequate energy and carbohydrates. Otherwise, you can trigger a primal drive to overeat. Once you reach the moment of excessive hunger, all intentions of moderate, conscious eating are fleeting and irrelevant. Learning to honor this first biological signal sets the stage for rebuilding trust with yourself and food.

A critical step to becoming an Intuitive Eater for Tim, a busy physician, was learning to honor his hunger. Tim dieted all through medical school while trying to keep up with a frenetic schedule working over eighty hours a week. He felt hungry most of the time, but ignored these signals because he was watching his weight. By midafternoon, his eating was out of control with snack attacks at the vending machine. His weight fluctuated with each dieting attempt (and failure). Not surprisingly, he felt low in energy most of the time.

Today, Tim has learned to pay attention to his biological signals of hunger and to honor them by taking the time to feed himself.

He knows now that if he doesn't listen to his growling stomach and eat breakfast before he leaves for work, he can't concentrate on what his patients are saying during their morning appointments. Tim has learned to *honor his hunger.*

As a result of becoming an Intuitive Eater, Tim feels full of energy throughout the day and is back to his college weight (maintaining a fifteen-pound weight loss). He has ended the cycles of restriction and overeating that plagued him for twenty years and feels confident that this futile cycle is gone forever.

PRINCIPLE 3:

MAKE PEACE WITH FOOD

Call a truce; stop the food fight! Give yourself unconditional permission to eat. If you tell yourself that you can't or shouldn't have a particular food, it can lead to intense feelings of deprivation that build into uncontrollable cravings and, often, bingeing. When you finally "give in" to your forbidden foods, eating will be experienced with such intensity, it usually results in Last Supper overeating and overwhelming guilt.

Nancy is a waitress whose battleground was a gourmet restaurant offering an array of delicious, rich foods. Before becoming an Intuitive Eater, Nancy would valiantly refrain from all of the tempting foods available at the restaurant. She would leave each night, physically tired and with haunting visions of the foods she shouldn't have. Her restraint was consistent, until making her first appointment. Suddenly in the week prior to her coming in, all she wanted to do was eat. And eat, she did!

Nancy experienced the Last Supper effect that accompanies intense food deprivation. She had an eating backlash from not allowing herself to touch her favorite foods. Nancy believed that any nutritionist would confirm that she had to give up these foods for good *and* follow a rigid meal plan. She acknowledged feeling scared and angry about her future food loss and automatically went into a phase of overeating, especially foods that she perceived would be forbidden forever.

Now that Nancy is an Intuitive Eater, she eats whatever appeals to her at the restaurant (and elsewhere). She no longer restricts the foods she likes, nor does she overeat and feel guilty. She discovered that some of the foods that looked wonderful didn't even taste good! Nancy has *made peace with food*, and loves the freedom that comes with it.

PRINCIPLE 4:

CHALLENGE THE FOOD POLICE

Scream a loud "No" to thoughts in your head that declare you're "good" for eating under 1,000 calories or "bad" because you ate a piece of chocolate cake. The Food Police monitor the unreasonable rules that dieting has created. The police station is housed deep in your psyche and its loudspeaker shouts negative barbs, hopeless phrases, and guilt-provoking indictments. Chasing the Food Police away is a critical step in returning to Intuitive Eating.

As an adolescent, Linda had been a competitive track sprinter and went on to qualify for the Olympic trials. Linda's coach had been a strong influence in her life, and to this day, her coach's voice reverberates, "To be competitive, you must diet to get rid of body fat." She can also hear her mother's voice chiming in about which foods are "good" and "bad."

Years of weight fluctuations resulted from obeying the monotonous dieting tapes droning in her head. These inner tapes culminated from her well-meaning coach and numerous diets, only to be reinforced with negative messages that her mother doled out. Linda's Food Police strengthened with each diet, each coaching admonishment, and each motherly chastisement.

Linda's breakthrough came when she discovered how to *challenge the Food Police*. Linda learned to talk back to the inner critical voices that tried to restrict her food choices. She learned to give herself nurturing messages and make nonjudgmental decisions about her eating.

The voice of the Intuitive Eater was allowed to re-emerge once the Food Police were silenced. Linda is now guilt-free about her eating, and her weight has stabilized at its natural level without dieting.

PRINCIPLE 5:

FEEL YOUR FULLNESS

Listen for the body signals that tell you you are no longer hungry. Observe the signs that show you're comfortably full. Pause in the middle of eating and ask yourself how the food tastes, and what your current fullness level is.

Jackie was a party girl. She loved to go out to eat with her friends every night after work and felt that weekends were not complete without a party. Jackie loved life and loved to eat. But she also didn't know how to stop eating when she began to feel full. (Rather, she often did not recognize feeling full until she was uncomfortably satiated, stuffed.) The morning after each social event she made the same vow: "I never want to eat again. I feel sick and stuffed and bloated, and I hate this roll around my middle."

Learning to *feel fullness* was a key element in Jackie's journey to Intuitive Eating. She began to pay attention to the transition from an empty stomach to a slightly full stomach. She soon learned to sense the signals of fullness that started to emerge in the midst of her meals.

It was easier for Jackie to honor her body's satiety signals when she truly knew she could eat again if hungry (even within the hour), and eat her favorite foods. (What starving person would stop at comfortable fullness if he thought he *was* never going to eat again, or have access to a particular food?) Jackie made an interesting observation during one of her out-of-town parties, while feeding alley cats: The starving alley cat will eat until the bowl is licked clean, unlike finicky cats—they know they will be fed again, so they can easily turn up their tails and leave food in their dish. Finicky cats can honor fullness because they know they will eat again.

Jackie also discovered that by honoring satiety signals and pushing her plate away (when *she* was ready) she was showing more respect for herself. After becoming an Intuitive Eater, Jackie felt that she had it all. She could still go out with her friends whenever she liked, and she could wake up the next morning feeling great!

PRINCIPLE 6:

DISCOVER THE SATISFACTION FACTOR

The Japanese have the wisdom to keep pleasure as one of their goals of healthy living. In our fury to be thin and healthy, we often overlook one of the most basic gifts of existence—the pleasure and satisfaction that can be found in the eating experience. When you eat what you really want, in an environment that is inviting, the pleasure you derive will be a powerful force in helping you feel satisfied and content. By providing this experience for yourself, you will find that it takes much less food to decide you've had "enough."

Denise is a movie production assistant who was surrounded by a variety of "forbidden" foods each day when she went to the set. Instead of giving herself permission to eat what she really wanted, she would ignore her preference signals. If she wanted french fries, she would nobly substitute an austere baked potato, unadorned. If cookies beckoned, she'd settle for fruit. Rather than stopping at her substitute food choice, however, she'd continue to seek out food after food, trying to find satisfaction in lowfat foods. Denise couldn't understand why she wasn't losing weight, especially since she was choosing only lean foods.

Once Denise realized that all of these alternate food choices were only fillers, that none of them led her to feel satisfied, she decided to experiment: Eat what she was craving. She was delighted to find that not only did she get true pleasure from the food, but she stopped eating as soon as she finished the portion—sometimes even leaving some behind! She was satisfied and content not needing to seek out a replacement for her "phantom food." Denise *discovered the satisfaction factor* in eating. She eats far less than ever before, and has lost the weight she struggled with for years. Denise experienced the benefits of our motto, "If you don't love it, don't eat it, and if you love it, savor it."

PRINCIPLE 7:

COPE WITH YOUR EMOTIONS WITHOUT USING FOOD

Find ways to comfort, nurture, distract, and resolve your issues without using food. Anxiety, loneliness, boredom, and anger are emotions we all experience throughout life. Each has its own trigger, and each has its own appeasement. Food won't fix any of these feelings. It may comfort for the short term, distract from the pain, or even numb you into a food hangover. But food won't solve the problem. If anything, eating for an emotional hunger will only make you feel worse in the long run. You'll ultimately have to deal with the source of the emotion, as well as the discomfort of overeating.

Marsha was a writer who did most of her work at home. She loved her work, but sometimes found that she would have mini periods of writer's block. To relieve her tension about finding the right word to put on the computer, she would visit the kitchen many times during the day to get a snack. Marsha was *using* food to help her get her work done.

Lisa was a fourteen-year-old who would come home after school and plop herself down in front of the TV with a bag of potato chips. Lisa was *using* food to procrastinate doing her homework.

Cynthia's children were grown; she had an illness that depleted her energy, not allowing her to go to work, and her husband didn't pay much attention to her. Cynthia found food to keep her occupied when she was bored and to soothe her lonely soul.

Using food to cope with emotions comes in degrees of intensity. For some, food is simply a means of distraction from boring activities or a filler for empty times. For others, it can be the *only* comfort they have to get through a painful life.

Before becoming Intuitive Eaters, Marsha, Lisa, and Cynthia were coping with their problems by using food as a distracter, comforter, and calmer. But they soon learned to savor the foods they had chosen, to eat in an inviting environment, and to honor their biological hungers. Increased gratifying eating experiences allowed each to let go of using food as a coping mechanism. They also offered clarity—it was easier to distinguish an eating urge from an emotional urge.

These women discovered that food never tasted as good or was as satisfying when they weren't really hungry, or hadn't figured out what they really wanted to eat, or bolted food down without respecting fullness. Marsha, Lisa, and Cynthia learned to *cope without using food* and to find appropriate outlets for their emotions. Now they save their eating for the times it gives them true satisfaction, and eat far smaller quantities of food.

PRINCIPLE 8:

RESPECT YOUR BODY

Accept your genetic blueprint. Just as a person with a shoe size of eight would not expect realistically to squeeze into a size six, it is equally futile (and uncomfortable) to have a similar expectation about body size. Respect your body so you can feel better about who you are. It's hard to reject the diet mentality if you are unrealistic and overly critical of your body shape.

One of the most important goals that Andrea had while working toward becoming an Intuitive Eater, was to *respect her body*. She was fifty years old, had given birth to four children, and was a valuable member of the community. Her body had gotten her through childbirth, traveling, working, and exercise. It was a body to respect rather than belittle. Yet, Andrea spent many of her waking hours criticizing her body and remembering the days when she was younger and thinner. The more she made negative comments to herself, the more despair she felt. She would turn to food when she wasn't hungry to console herself for her misery. She also found herself overeating as a way to punish herself for looking so "bad."

Once Andrea stopped comparing herself to every other woman she knew and started to respect and honor her body, she began to eat less and to take better care of herself. Andrea became an Intuitive Eater, lost weight, took pride in her achievements, and stopped trying to have the "perfect" body.

Janie, a twenty-five-year-old publicist, also played the "body-check" game. Every time she was at a party, she silently compared herself to other women, only to feel that she was the heaviest woman in attendance. Ironically, Janie had a very fit build, but felt mortified each time and would vow that night to begin a diet the next day. Only when Janie began to focus on respecting her body and its inner cues rather than external forces (what other people look like, what other people are doing) did she make a significant breakthrough.

PRINCIPLE 9:

EXERCISE—FEEL THE DIFFERENCE

Forget militant exercise. Just get active and *feel* the difference. Shift your focus to how it feels to move your body, rather than the calorie-burning effect of exercise. If you focus on how you feel from working out, such as energized, it can make the difference between rolling out of bed for a brisk morning walk or hitting the snooze alarm. If when you wake up your only goal is to lose weight, it's usually not a motivating factor in that moment of time.

Miranda had all the accoutrements of a regular exerciser—a membership in a gym, a stationary bike at home, athletic clothes and shoes. There was just one problem—she was *not* exercising. Miranda was burned out. She had tried almost as many new exercise programs as she had diets. It was a vicious cycle—begin a diet and simultaneously begin working out, then quit both the diet and the exercise. That was precisely the problem. Miranda never really felt the pleasure of exercise, of moving her body. Part of the problem was that when she was underfeeding her body (dieting), she had little energy, if any, to exercise—and that *does not feel good.* Consequently, exercising was always a struggle. It was only the initial enthusiasm and momentum of the diet that would carry her through a monotonous workout. But because the dieting was short-lived, so too was the exercise.

When Miranda began feeding her body (by *honoring her hunger*), she felt better and entertained the idea of beginning a walking program. She discovered that by reframing the purpose of exercise from a weight loss tool to feeling good, she began to actually enjoy walking. For the first time in her life Miranda is consistently exercising and *enjoying* it. She also knows that she will continue to be consistent because she enjoys the pay-off, which includes feeling better about herself.

PRINCIPLE 10:

HONOR YOUR HEALTH—GENTLE NUTRITION

Make food choices that honor your health and taste buds while making you feel good. Remember that you don't have to eat a perfect diet to be healthy. You will not suddenly get a nutrient deficiency or gain weight from one snack, one meal, or one day of eating. It's what you eat consistently over time that matters. Progress, not perfection, is what counts.

Louise, like so many of our clients, had dieted all her life. She had been enlightened by the antidieting movement and was ahead of the game with a reject-dieting mentality. But Louise had been meticulously counting fat grams like a dieter counting calories, so in essence, she was still dieting. She was using nutrition information militantly to keep herself in check. Her food choices were primarily fat-free foods; they were safe and healthy, she reasoned. Yet, Louise couldn't understand why she was still bingeing. When Louise realized that she was using nutrition as a dieting weapon, rather than as an ally for health, she began to change the way she chose her foods. Louise honored her taste buds and listened to her body with respect to how food made her feel. When Louise was finally able to relax her eating, to eat with less rigidity, she discovered that it was possible to honor both the pleasure of taste and her health. And by doing this she was more satisfied with eating, her binges ceased, and she was able to attain her natural healthy weight.

A PROCESS WITH GREAT REWARDS

All of the clients mentioned in the above examples had been dissatisfied with their relationship with food and their bodies. Each had tried either formal or informal dieting and had felt failure and despair. By learning the principles of Intuitive Eating and putting them to work, each found a deepening of the quality of life and resolution about eating. You can too!

Chapter Four

Awakening the Intuitive Eater: Stages

The journey to Intuitive Eating is like taking a cross-country hiking trip. Before you even strap on your hiking boots you want to know what to expect during your journey. While a road map is helpful, it doesn't describe what you'll need to know to be adequately prepared, such as trail conditions, climate, special sightseeing spots, what kind of clothes to wear, and so forth. The purpose of this chapter is to help you understand what to expect during your journey to Intuitive Eating.

Whether it's hiking or relearning a more satisfying eating style, you will go through many stages along the way. The amount of time that you need to stay in any particular stage is variable and highly individualized. For example, traversing new hiking trails depends on how physically fit you are, how you deal with fear of new trails, how much time you have to hike, and the availability of hiking trails. Similarly, your journey back to Intuitive Eating depends on how long you've been dieting, how strongly entrenched your diet thinking is, how long you've been using food to cope with life, how willing you are to trust yourself, and how willing you are to make weight loss a secondary goal and learning to become an Intuitive Eater the primary goal.

Sometimes, you'll move back and forth among the stages. If you accept that this is a normal part of the process, it will help you to keep going without feeling that you are backsliding or not making progress.

Consider this scenario: You are on a hiking trail, and encounter a fork in the road that is hard to decipher with your trail map. Do you go to the right or left? You ponder for a while and decide to go left. While walking, you spot something you've never seen before, a bright green caterpillar shimmying up a purple flower. A few steps ahead, you discover an unusual bird. But a few steps beyond these glories of nature is a big boulder signaling that you chose the wrong path. You turn around, go back to the fork, and take the other path. Was this detour a waste of time? No. Similarly, on the path to Intuitive Eating, you will take many turns and experiment with new thoughts and behaviors. You may even find that after making noticeable progress, you go back to old ways that are uncomfortable and unfulfilling. But, like taking the "wrong" path on the scenic hiking trail, you'll discover that excursions into old eating patterns can be used as learning experiences. (Most hikers would not chide themselves for being unsure of which path to take; instead, they'd be grateful for the discoveries of nature that a blocked path offered.) It's important to be kind to yourself and appreciate the learning that comes out of the experience. This process involves coming from a place of curiosity, rather than a place of judgment, so whatever you do, don't beat yourself up mentally!

Intuitive Eating is very different from dieting. Dieters usually get frustrated when they don't follow the diet path exactly as prescribed. We have seen many a chronic dieter merely take a wrong turn at one meal, be critical for that mistake, and "blow" the diet for that day or weekend or even longer!

Keep in mind that the journey to Intuitive Eating is a *process* complete with ups and downs, unlike dieting, where the common expectation is linear progress (losing a certain amount of weight in a specific time period).

Take a look at the graph comparing dieting and Intuitive Eating. Note how the graph for Intuitive Eating resembles a tracking table for the stock market. The road to Intuitive Eating is like investing in a long-term mutual fund. Over time, there will be return on the investment in spite of the daily fluctuations of the stock market. It is normal and expected. How ironic that we have been taught that, in economics, the day-to-day changes in the stock market are normal and there is seldom a quick get-rich fix, yet in the weight-loss business "get thin fast" is often seen as the only goal for success. Keep in mind Webster's definition of *process*: "a continuing development involving many changes," and "a particular method of doing something, generally involving a number of steps or operations."

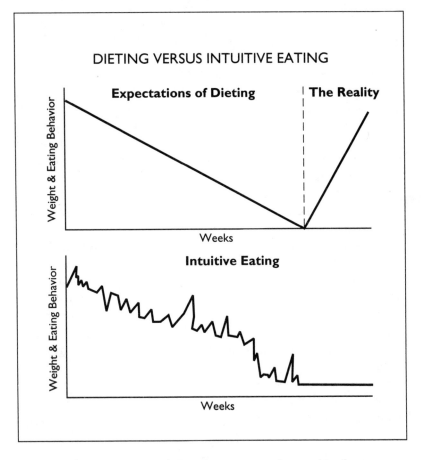

As with any process, it's important to stay focused in the present, and grow from the many experiences you will encounter. If, however, you focus on the end result (which for most people is the amount of pounds lost), it can make you feel overwhelmed and discouraged, and end up sabotaging the process. Instead, if you acknowledge small changes along the way and value the learning experiences (which can be frustrating), it will help you stay on the Intuitive Eating path and move forward. Once you truly become an Intuitive Eater, your body will return to its natural weight level and remain there. For many people, that means losing weight.

To find out if you are a good candidate for weight loss, ask yourself the following: Have you routinely eaten beyond your comfortable fullness level? Do you routinely overeat when you're getting ready for your next diet (knowing there will be a lot of foods you won't be allowed to eat)? Do you overeat as a coping mechanism in difficult times or to fill up time when you're bored? Have you also been resistant to exercise? Do you only exercise when you diet? Do you skip meals or wait to eat until you're ravenously hungry, only to find that you overeat when you finally do eat? Do you feel guilty, either when you overeat or when you eat a "bad food," which results in more overeating? If you answered "yes" to some or all of these questions, then it's likely that you will be able to return to your natural healthy weight as a result of this process.

Once you've given up dieting forever, you'll find yourself eating far less food and wanting to exercise regularly. You'll find that your body feels so much better when your stomach isn't overfilled, when your muscles are toned and your heart is fit. If you *focus on how you feel as the goal, rather than on weight loss*, you'll find, ironically, that you can't help but lose weight. If, instead, you continue to focus on weight loss as the goal, you'll get tied up in the old diet-mentality thinking and find that permanent weight loss is like a carrot dangling on that stick in front of you—you're forever dieting without reaching the mark.

Over the years, we have seen that our patients go through a five-stage progression in learning how to become Intuitive Eaters. The following section will help you get an idea of what to expect in your own personal journey.

STAGE ONE:
READINESS—HITTING DIET BOTTOM

This is where most people begin. You are painfully aware that every attempt to lose weight has ended in failure. You are tired of valuing each day based on whether the scale is up or down a pound or two (or if you've overeaten the day before). You think and worry about food all the time. You talk the restrictive food talk—"If only I didn't have to watch my weight, I could eat that," or "I had two cookies— I was really bad today."

Your weight could fall into one of three patterns: It's higher than ever before; you are stuck at a plateau and pounds won't budge; or while not greatly overweight, you gain and lose five or ten pounds as frequently and rapidly as your laundry gets dirty and then clean again.

You have lost touch with biological hunger and satiety signals. You have forgotten what you really like to eat and instead eat what you think you "should" eat. Your relationship with food has developed a negative tone and you dread eating the foods you love because you're afraid it will be hard to stop. When you give in to the temptation of forbidden foods, it's not unusual to overeat because you feel guilty. Yet you sincerely vow you will never eat them again.

It's not unusual to find that you eat to comfort, distract, or even numb yourself from your feelings. If that's the case, you will sense that the quality of your life has been clouded by obsessional thinking about food and by mindless eating.

Your body image is negative—you don't like the way you look and feel in your body, and self-respect is lessened. You have learned from your own experience that dieting does not work–you have hit diet bottom and feel stuck, frustrated, and discouraged.

This stage continues until you decide that you are unhappy eating and living this way—and you are ready to do something about it. Your first thoughts may veer toward finding a new diet to solve your problems. But almost immediately, you realize that you just can't do that one ever again. If this is where you find yourself, then you are ready for the process that will bring you back to eating intuitively.

STAGE TWO: EXPLORATION—CONSCIOUS LEARNING AND PURSUIT OF PLEASURE

This is a stage of exploration and discovery. You will go through a phase of *hyperconsciousness* to help reacquaint yourself with your intuitive signals: hunger, taste preferences, and satiety.

This stage is a lot like learning how to drive a car. For the novice driver, just getting the car out of the driveway requires a lot of conscious thinking, complete with a mental checklist: Put the key in the ignition, make sure the gear is in park or neutral, turn on the engine, check the rearview mirror, remove the hand brake, and so forth. This hyperconsciousness is necessary to lock in all of the steps needed just to get that car in first gear! In the same sense, you will be zooming in on details of eating that have evolved without such focused thinking. (But this is necessary to reclaim the Intuitive Eater in you.)

It may seem awkward and uncomfortable, even obsessive. However, hyperconsciousness is different from obsessive thinking. Obsessive thinking is pervasive and is characterized by worry. It fills your mind during most of the day and keeps you from thinking of much else. Hyperconsciousness is more specific. It zooms in when you have a thought about food, but goes away when the eating experience is over. And just like the steps required to drive a car become autopilot for the experienced driver, Intuitive Eating will eventually be experienced without this initial awkwardness.

You may feel that you are in a hyperconscious state much of the time during this stage. This may feel uncomfortable at first and perhaps even strange. Remember, much of your previous eating was either mostly unconscious or diet-directed.

In this stage, you'll begin to *make peace with food* by giving yourself unconditional permission to eat. This part may feel scary and you may choose to move slowly (within your comfort level). You will learn to get rid of guilt-induced eating and begin to discover the importance of the satisfaction factor with food. The more satisfied you are when eating, the less you will think about food when you are not hungry—you will no longer be on the prowl.

You will experiment with foods that you have not eaten for a long time. This includes sorting out your *true* food likes and dislikes. You may even discover that you don't like the taste of some of the foods you've been dreaming of! (Keep in mind that years of dieting, or eating what you "should," only serve to disconnect you from your internal eating drive and true food preferences.)

You will learn to *honor your hunger* and recognize your body signals that indicate the many degrees of hunger. You will learn to separate these biological signals from the emotional signals that might also trigger eating.

In this stage, you may find that you are eating larger quantities of foods than your body needs. It will be difficult to *respect your fullness* at this stage, because you need time to experiment with the quantity it takes to satisfy a deprived palate. It also takes time for you to develop trust with food again and know that it's truly okay to eat. How can you honor fullness if you are not completely sure it's okay to eat a particular food, or if you fear it won't be there tomorrow?

During this stage, weight gain usually ceases or is limited to just a few pounds. If you have been using food emotionally, you may find that you will begin to *feel* your feelings and may experience discomfort, sadness, or even depression at times.

The bulk of your eating may be in foods that are heavier in fat and sugar than you've been accustomed to—although you may have been eating large quantities of these foods secretly or with guilt. *The way you eat during this stage will not be the pattern that you will establish or want for a lifetime.* You will notice that your nutritional balance is off kilter and you may not feel physically on top of things during this time. This is all normal and expected. You must let yourself go through this stage for as long as you need. Remember, you are making up for years of deprivation, negative self-talk, and guilt. You are rebuilding positive food experiences, like a strand of pearls. Each food experience, like each pearl, may seem insignificant, but collectively they make a difference.

STAGE THREE: CRYSTALLIZATION

In this stage you will experience the first awakenings of the Intuitive Eating style that has always been a part of you, but was buried under the debris of dieting. When you enter this stage, much of the exploration work from the previous stage begins to crystallize and feels like solid behavior change. Your thoughts about food are no longer obsessional. You hardly need to maintain the hyperconsciousness about eating that was originally needed. Consequently, your eating decisions don't require quite as much directed thought. Instead, you find that your food choices and responses to biological signals are mainly intuitive.

You have a greater sense of trust—both in your right to choose what you really want to eat and in the fact that your biological signals are dependable. You are more comfortable with your food choices and will start to notice increased satisfaction at your meals.

At this point, you *honor your hunger* most of the time, and it's easier to discern what you feel like eating when you are hungry. You continue to *make peace with food.*

What feels new in this stage is that it's easier to pause in the midst of your meal to consciously gauge how much your stomach is filling up. You will be able to take note of your fullness and respect the presence of that signal, although you may find that you often eat beyond the fullness mark. Just like when an archer takes aim at a new target, it often requires shooting many arrows before learning how to reach the bull's-eye. You may still be choosing heavier foods most of the time, but you will find that you don't need as much of them to satisfy you.

If you've been an emotionally cued eater, you'll become quite adept at separating biological hunger signals from emotional hunger. Because of this clarity, more often than not, you will be experiencing your feelings and finding ways to comfort and distract yourself without the use of food.

Some weight loss may occur during this stage, especially if you have quite a bit of weight to lose. If not, you'll see that you're maintaining your weight, rather than bouncing up and down. But more important than weight loss at this stage, is the sense of well-being and empowerment that begins to take place. You won't feel helpless and hopeless anymore. You will begin to respect your body and understand that it is where it's at as a result of the dieting mentality, rather than lack of willpower.

STAGE FOUR:
THE INTUITIVE EATER AWAKENS

By the time you reach this stage, all the work you have been doing culminates in a comfortable, free-flowing eating style. You consistently choose what you really want to eat when you are hungry. Because you know that you can have more food, of your choosing, whenever you are hungry, it's easy to stop eating when you feel comfortably full.

You will begin to find that you choose lighter and healthier foods, not because you think you should, but because you *feel* better physically when you eat this way. The urgent need to prove to yourself that you can have heavier foods will have diminished. You truly know and trust that these once forbidden foods will always be there, and if you really want to eat them, you can—so they lose their alluring quality. Chocolate starts to take on the same emotional connotation as a peach. You won't need to test yourself anymore, and your deprivation backlash with food will be gone.

When you do choose heavier foods, you will get great pleasure, and feel satisfied with a much smaller quantity than ever before, and without guilt.

If coping with your feelings has been difficult for you, you will be less afraid to experience them, and become more adept at sitting with them. Finding healthy alternatives to distract and comfort yourself when necessary will become natural for you.

Your food talk and self talk will be positive and noncritical. Your peace pact with food is firmly established and you will have released any conflict or left-over guilt about food choices that you have carried around.

You will have stopped being angry with your body and making disrespectful comments about it. You will respect it and accept that there are many different sizes and shapes in the world. At this point, weight loss will become more evident and your body will be on its way to approaching its natural weight.

STAGE FIVE:
THE FINAL STAGE—TREASURE THE PLEASURE

At this point, your Intuitive Eater has been reclaimed. You will trust your body's intuitive abilities—it will be easy to *honor your hunger* and *respect your fullness*. Finally, you will feel no guilt about your food choices or quantities. Because you feel good about your relationship to food and treasure the pleasure that eating now gives you, you will discard unsatisfying eating situations and unappealing foods.

You will want to experience eating in the most optimal of conditions and not taint it with emotional distress. You will feel an inner conviction to give up using food to cope with emotional situations, if that has been your habit. You will find that you would much rather deal with your feelings or distract yourself from them with anything other than food, when emotions become too overwhelming.

Because your eating style has become a source of pleasure rather than an affliction, you will experience nutrition and exercise in a different way. The *burden* of exercise will be removed and exercising will begin to look enticing to you. Exercise will no longer be used as a driving force to burn more calories; rather, you become committed to exercise as a way to *feel* better, physically and mentally. Likewise, nutrition will no longer be another mechanism for making you feel bad about the way you eat; instead, it becomes a path to feeling as physically good and healthy as you can.

When you reach the final stage, your weight will naturally decrease (if you had weight to lose) to a place that is comfortable and appropriate for your height. If your weight was already normal, you will find that you can maintain it with no effort and will be rid of the emotional ups and downs that accompany the restriction/ overeating cycles.

At last, you will feel empowered and protected from outside forces telling you what and how much to eat, and how your body should look. You will feel free of the burden of dieting. And you will be an Intuitive Eater once again.

YOU CAN DO IT!

These stages and the changes that occur with your eating and thoughts may seem impossible. Or, they might seem too scary. For example, the thought of giving yourself unconditional permission to eat may seem terrifying—and you might fear that you will never stop eating and will gain even more weight. The remainder of the book explains in great detail how to implement each principle, why it is needed and the rationale behind it. You will also find how other chronic dieters became Intuitive Eaters and how it changed their lives. By the time you finish reading this book you will know that you too can become an Intuitive Eater, and stop the madness of dieting.

Chapter Five

Reject the Diet Mentality

Throw out the diet books and magazine articles that offer you the false hope of losing weight quickly, easily, and permanently. Get angry at the lies that have led you to feel as if you were a failure every time a new diet stopped working and you gained back all of the weight. If you allow even one small hope to linger that a new and better diet might be lurking around the corner, it will prevent you from being free to rediscover Intuitive Eating.

If you're like most clients we see, the idea of *not* dieting can be scary, even when you know that you can't choke down one more diet plan or drink. It's normal to feel panicky about letting go of dieting, especially when the world around you is on some diet. It has been the only tool you have known to lose weight, albeit temporarily.

Hitting diet bottom is a paralyzing feeling—damned if you diet and damned if you don't. Many of our clients feel stuck between two conflicting fears: "If I continue dieting, I'll ruin my metabolism and gain weight," and "If I stop dieting, I'll gain *more* weight." Other common fears that we hear are:

FEAR: If I stop dieting, I won't stop eating.

REALITY: Dieting often *triggers* overeating. Of course it's hard to stop eating when you've been undereating and restricting food; it's a normal response to starvation. (You'll hear more about that in the next chapter!) But once your body learns, and trusts, that you will not be starving it anymore through dieting, the intense drive for eating will decrease.

FEAR: I don't know how to eat when I'm not dieting.

REALITY: When you banish diets and become an Intuitive Eater, you will be eating in response to inner signals, which will guide your eating. This is like learning how to swim for the first time. The feeling of being surrounded by water can be terrifying to the novice swimmer, especially when totally submerged. Similarly, being surrounded by food can be terrifying to the chronic dieter who is learning how to eat again. But you will not learn how to swim by merely standing at the edge of the pool (even while believing that learning how to swim is a good thing). First you begin by getting your feet wet and learning how to breathe in the water. Eventually, you will put your head in the water when you are ready—and you get more comfortable.

FEAR: I will be out of control.

REALITY: You will feel in control through Intuitive Eating, rather than relying on external factors and authority figures whom you're bound to defy. You will learn to listen to and honor your inner cues, both physical and emotional—a powerful ability.

THE DIET VOID

For many people, dieting has been a way to cope with life, from filling up time, to exercising a semblance of control. Think of the times in your life in which you started a diet. How often did your diets coincide with difficult times or transitions? It's not unusual to begin a diet during the following life transitions: passing from childhood to adolescence, leaving home, marrying, starting a new job, or experiencing marital difficulties. While dieting may have been futile, it offered excitement and hope—the exhilaration of quick weight loss and the excitement of watching the scale inch downwards, the hope that this diet will be it. It's similar to going to a hairstylist for a new cut, with the expectation that it will revolutionize the way you look and feel about yourself and maybe change your life. But when you say good-bye to the thrill and excitement of dieting, you'll also be letting go of the false hope and disappointments from dieting.

There is a social element to dieting that you may miss, *diet bonding*. When you decide to give up dieting, you might be surprised how often new diets and dieting are the topic of conversation at parties, with friends, at work—and now you won't be playing *that* game. It might feel like a must-see movie everyone is talking about, only you haven't seen it and have no plans to view it either. You might feel a little left out, detached. Remember, as long as there is money to be made, there will always be a new gimmick or diet for a quick-weight-loss fix. Just recently the manufacturer of a product called "Sleepers Diet" claimed to help people attain greater weight loss while sleeping. Talk about dreaming! The manufacturer was fined by the FTC for making unsubstantiated claims. But people still shelled out the money for this new gimmick.

THE ONE-LAST-DIET TRAP

The initial step to becoming an Intuitive Eater is to reject the diet mentality. Yet even when you come to terms with the futility and harm that dieting unleashes on the body and mind, it can be a difficult first step, as described in a letter below from a client, Lisa:

> *I have been in the dieting dilemma all my life. Every diet I've ever been on has worked for me, at least what I thought of as worked. Worked in the past was losing a certain number of pounds, never considering the reality of regaining the weight plus more with each and every diet I went on. At age thirty-six, I came to a point in my life where I was dieted-out. I knew there had to be another way. Yet my first thought was to let myself find one more diet for the last time and I would make a promise to myself to never gain the weight back through a change in lifestyle.*

Lisa's letter represents a common conflict of chronic dieters. You've hit diet bottom, you know dieting doesn't work but you're desperate—just one more diet, just this time, "I'll be good." And so begins the familiar chronic dieter's plea: Just let me lose the weight now, and *after* I lose the weight, I'll figure it out. But as long as you cling to a small hope that a quick little diet will turn your weight around, or jump-start you into a new person, you won't be free from the tyranny of dieting. Giving in to just-one-more-diet is one of the biggest traps, because it doesn't face the reality—diets do not work. So how could another diet truly be part of the solution?

Jackie, another client, had been dieting all of her life since the age of twelve. By the time she came in, Jackie thought she was ready to give up dieting. Jackie made a lot of progress in three months, which for her was stabilized weight. For the first time, she began to have a normal relationship with food rather than constant food worry and obsession. But she wanted to take a break from our work together. Five months later Jackie called, she needed to come back desperately. Jackie said she "finally got it." She knew once and for all that dieting creates *more* problems. Jackie revealed that during our initial work she had secretly hoped a little diet was all she needed. She thought losing some quick pounds would allow her to work on her "real food issues" without worrying about her body, and then she would have more patience. It was part of her reason for leaving.

When Jackie left, she dabbled with two serious quickie diets, which resulted in disaster. She lost ten pounds quickly (through juice fasting and intense exercise), and got excited. She was so "motivated" that she was sure if she lost another ten pounds through a different food-combining diet, her problems would be over. Jackie couldn't have been further from the truth. She became more obsessed with food and began bingeing. Not only did she gain back every pound, but she got *heavier*, became more frustrated, and had less trust in herself with food.

Every diet is like a Hoola Hoop flung onto your body. At first it's effortless to keep the hoop in motion. But eventually massive layers of Hoola Hoops disrupt normal rhythm and become binding. You cannot rotate the Hoola Hoop—you can't even move. To get yourself out of the last-chance diet trap, you need to come to terms with the fact that dieting doesn't work and can in fact be harmful. Perhaps you're inclined to argue however, that you'll feel better about yourself when you lose the weight. But studies have shown that improvements in psychological well-being associated with weight loss are just as temporary as the pounds lost and regained. The "good feelings" diminish with regained weight, and existing issues of self-worth and general psychological function return to the original levels when weight is regained.

PSEUDO-DIETING

Many of our clients state, "I've given up dieting," but they still have trouble shaking the diet mentality. They may be physically off a diet, but the dieting thoughts remain. The problem is that dieting thoughts usually translate into dietlike behaviors, which becomes pseudo-dieting or unconscious dieting. Consequently, these clients will still suffer the side effects of dieting, but it's much harder to spot (and then they really feel out of control with their eating). Pseudo-dieting behaviors are not usually apparent to the person engaged in them. Keep in mind that eating is so universal, it's hard to be objective. It can be difficult to find the loopholes in your own eating mentality/ behavior if you don't know what you are looking for. To the surprise of our clients, they often don't discover that they have been pseudo-dieting until *together* we review their eating history. Here are some examples of pseudo-dieting:

• *Meticulously counting fat grams* is the modern version of counting calories. While knowing fat grams has its merits, the act of counting fat grams to control weight is really no different from counting calories. Many of our chronic dieters are pros at rationing their fat grams for the day—and they are stuck.

• *Eating only "safe" foods*. This usually means sticking with fat-free and/or low-calorie foods, beyond counting fat grams. For example, one client would not eat any food that listed more than one gram of fat on the food label, regardless of what her total fat and calorie intake for the day was. Remember, however, that one food, one meal, or one day will not make or break your health or your weight.

• *Eating only at certain times of the day*, whether or not you are hungry, is a common leftover habit from dieting, especially *not* eating after a certain time of night, such as after 6:00 P.M. Reality check: Our bodies do not punch time clocks; we do not suddenly turn off our need for energy. This can especially be a problem for a dieter who exercises after work, comes home late—around 7:30 P.M.—and decides it's too late to eat for fear that the fat meter is in high gear. While it is reasonable to not want to go to bed on a full stomach, to deny a hungry body *any* food or energy is unreasonable.

• *Paying penance for eating "bad" foods* such as cookies, cheesecake, or ice cream. The penalty can include skipping the next meal, eating less, vowing to be "good" tomorrow, or doing *extra* exercise.

• *Cutting back on food*, especially when feeling fat or when a special event such as a wedding or class reunion comes up. While cutting back sounds innocent enough, it's amazing how often this gets acted out in the form of unconscious *undereating*. Remember, undereating usually triggers overeating.

• *Pacifying hunger by drinking coffee or diet soda*. This is a common dieting trick to assuage hunger pangs without eating or calories.

• *Limiting carbohydrates*. We are struck by the number of clients who profess they know of the importance of consuming this fuel, yet eat an *inadequate* amount of carbohydrates, such as bread, pasta, and rice, because they are afraid they will gain weight.

• *Putting on a "false food face" in public*, eating only what is "proper" in front of other people. One client, Alice, ate an enjoyable meal with friends. When the dessert tray came around she really wanted a piece of pie, but fought the urge because she wanted to appear to be a healthy, weight-conscious eater. However, on her way home, the urge for the pie swelled into an uncontrollable craving. Alice stopped at the store, bought a whole pie, and ate one fourth of it, which was *more* than she would have eaten had she honored her true food preference earlier! This social dieting behavior of putting on a false food face backfired (and it often does).

• *Competing with someone else who is dieting*—feeling obligated to be equally virtuous (if not more). Because dieting is viewed as a virtuous trait in our society, it is not unusual that you would get sucked into appearing virtuous. This can easily occur when friends, family, or a significant other is dieting.

• *Second-guessing or judging what you deserve to eat* based on what you've eaten earlier in the day, rather than on hunger cues. One client, Sally, ate two large bowls of puffed rice cereal for breakfast after running for one hour. She thought that was too much food and later in the midmorning, did not allow herself to eat, although she was ravenous. Sally thought, "How could I be hungry only two hours after I ate a big breakfast?" The reality for Sally was that while her volume of food in the morning was larger than her norm, it was still *inadequate* for the amount of exercise she had done. Her body was trying to tell her, "I need more fuel," yet Sally felt guilty for being hungry. She also felt guilty for eating a big breakfast, until she realized that in actuality she had *undereaten*. Just because a meal or snack does not fit the "standard" portion size from your dieting days, it does not mean you are overeating!

* *Becoming a vegetarian only for the purpose of losing weight.* A vegetarian lifestyle can be a healthy way of eating and living, but if it is embraced with a diet mentality, it becomes merely another diet. For example, Karen began eating meatless to lose weight. But a month into her vegetarian eating she began craving meat. Never before had she experienced meat cravings! Karen realized she never really intended to become a vegetarian. She wasn't interested in vegetarian eating for health or ethical issues, only as a vehicle to lose weight, and so her diet backfired.

THE DIETER'S DILEMMA

Whether you are engaged in bona fide dieting or pseudo-dieting, any form of dieting is bound to lead to problems. The inherent futility of dieting is explained in the Dieter's Dilemma model created by psychologists John P. Foreyt and G. Ken Goodrick, shown on the next page. The Dieter's Dilemma is triggered with the desire to be thin, which leads to dieting. That's when the dilemma unfolds. Dieting increases cravings and urges for food. The dieter gives in to the craving, overeats, and eventually regains any lost weight. Then he is back to where he started, at the original weight—or higher. And once again the dieter has the desire to be thin ... and so another diet begins. The Dieter's Dilemma is perpetuated and gets worse with each turn of the cycle. The dieter gets heavier and feels more out of control with eating.

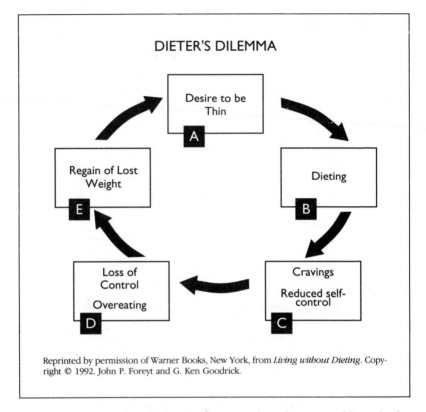

DIETER'S DILEMMA

Reprinted by permission of Warner Books, New York, from *Living without Dieting*. Copyright © 1992. John P. Foreyt and G. Ken Goodrick.

How do you break the futile Dieter's Dilemma? Although the antidieting movement is growing in popularity, there is always a new diet or program around the corner. You must simply make the decision to give up dieting.

HOW TO REJECT THE DIET MENTALITY

To let go of the dieting myth and the dieting mentality, our minds require a new frame of reference. In the best selling book *The 7 Habits of Highly Effective People*, author Stephen Covey popularized the concept of paradigm shifts. A paradigm is a model or frame of reference by which we perceive and understand the world. In the world of weight management, dieting is the cultural paradigm by which we attempt to control our weight. A paradigm shift is a break with tradition, with old ways of thinking, with old paradigms. We must change our paradigm to reject dieting; only then can we build a healthy relationship with food and our bodies.

While Covey's work is aimed at the business community, he hits upon an issue that rings true for chronic dieters. He believes that people are often drawn to remedy the problem without regard to the long-term implications of this "quick fix." He feels that this approach actually exacerbates the problem rather than permanently solving it. He points to the physical body as a prized asset that often is ruined, while one is on the race for rapid results and short-term benefits.

Here are the steps to beginning your paradigm shift and rejecting the diet mentality.

STEP I:
RECOGNIZE AND ACKNOWLEDGE
THE DAMAGE THAT DIETING CAUSES

There is a substantial amount of research on the harm that dieting causes. Acknowledge that the harm is real, and that continued dieting will only perpetuate your problems. Some of the key side effects gleaned from major studies are described below in two categories, biological and emotional. As you read, take a personal inventory and ask yourself which of the problems you are already experiencing. Recognizing that dieting is the problem will help you break through the cultural myth that diets work. Remember, *if dieting is the problem, how can it be part of the solution?*

Damage from Dieting: Biological and Health

In every century, famine and human starvation has existed. Sadly, this is true even today. Survival of the fittest in the past meant survival of the fattest—only those with adequate energy stores (fat) could survive a famine. Consequently, our bodies are still equipped in this modern age to combat starvation at the cellular level. As far as the body is concerned, dieting is a form of starvation, even though it's voluntary.

Chronic dieting has been shown to:

- *Teach the body to retain more fat when you start eating again.* Low-calorie diets double the enzymes that make and store fat in the body. This is a form of biological compensation to help the body store more energy, or fat, after dieting.

- *Slow the rate of weight loss* with each successive attempt to diet. This has been shown to be true in both rat and human studies.

- *Decrease metabolism.* Dieting triggers the body to become more efficient at utilizing calories by lowering the body's need for energy.

- *Increase binges and cravings.* Both humans and rats have been shown to overeat after chronic food restriction. Food restriction stimulates the brain to launch a cascade of cravings to eat *more*. After substantial weight loss, studies show that rats prefer eating more fat, while people have been shown to prefer foods both high in fat and sugar.

- *Increase risk of premature death and heart disease.* A thirty-two-year study of more than 3,000 men and women in the Framingham Heart Study has shown that *regardless of initial weight*, people whose weight repeatedly goes up and down—known as weight cycling or yo-yo dieting—have a higher overall death rate and twice the normal risk of dying from heart disease. These results were independent of cardiovascular risk factors, and held true regardless if a person was thin or obese. The harm from yo-yo dieting may be equal to the risks of staying obese.

Similarly, results of the Harvard Alumni Health Study show that people who lose and gain at least eleven pounds within a decade or so, don't live as long as those who maintain a stable weight.

- *Cause satiety cues to atrophy.* Dieters usually stop eating due to a self-imposed limit rather than inner cues of fullness. This, combined with skipping meals, can condition you to eat meals of increasingly larger size.

- *Cause body shape to change.* Yo-yo dieters who continually regain the lost weight tend to regain weight in the abdominal area. This type of fat storage increases the risk of heart disease.

Other documented side effects include headaches, menstrual irregularities, fatigue, dry skin, and hair loss.

Damage from Dieting: Psychological and Emotional

Psychological experts reported the following adverse effects at the landmark 1992 National Institutes of Health, Weight Loss and Control Conference:

- Dieting is linked to eating disorders.

- Dieting may cause stress or make the dieter more vulnerable to its effects.

- Independent of body weight itself, dieting is correlated with feelings of failure, lowered self-esteem, and social anxiety.

- The dieter is often vulnerable to loss of control over eating when violating "the rules" of the diet, whether there was an actual or *perceived* transgression of the diet! The mere perception of eating a forbidden food, regardless of actual calorie content, is enough to trigger overeating.

In a separate report, psychologists David Garner and Susan Wooley make a compelling case against the high cost of false hope from dieting. They conclude that:

- Dieting gradually erodes confidence and self-trust.

- Many obese individuals assume they could not have become obese unless they possessed some *fundamental character deficit.* Garner and Wooley argue that while many obese individuals may experience binge eating and depression, these psychological and behavioral symptoms are the *result of dieting.* But these overweight individuals easily interpret these symptoms as further evidence of an underlying problem. Yet, obese people do not have inordinate psychological disturbances compared to normal weight people.

STEP 2:
BE AWARE OF DIET-MENTALITY
TRAITS AND THINKING

The diet mentality surfaces in subtle forms, even when you decide to reject dieting. It's important to recognize common characteristics of the diet mentality; it will let you know if you are still playing the dieting game. Forget about willpower, being obedient, and failing. The general difference in the ways the dieter versus the nondieter views eating, exercise, and progress are summarized by a chart at the end of this chapter.

Forget Willpower. While no doctor would expect a patient to "will" blood pressure to normal levels, physicians frequently expect their overweight patients to "will" their weight loss by restricting their food, according to Susan Z. Yanovski, M.D. This is also a prevailing attitude among our clients and many Americans— all you need is willpower and a little self-control. In a 1993 Gallup poll, the most common obstacle to losing weight cited by women was willpower.

For example, Marilyn is a highly successful lawyer who climbed to the top of the corporate ladder. She credits determination, willpower, and self-discipline as being responsible for her success. Yet, when she tried to use these exemplary principles in her dieting attempts, she always failed. Whatever success she had achieved in her professional life was dulled by her sense of failure with eating.

Why was Marilyn able to be so disciplined in one area of her life but not in the other? The word "discipline" derives from the word "disciple." According to Stephen Covey's work, if you are a disciple to your own deep values that have an overriding purpose, it's likely that you'll have the *will* to carry them out. Marilyn believed deeply that writing exacting contracts and keeping immaculate records were requisites to building confidence with her clients and her law firm. But, somehow, hearing that bread was wrong on one diet and anything with sugar was wrong on another, did not engender the same kind of deep beliefs. Try as she might, she couldn't really believe that chocolate chip cookies were that evil!

Willpower can be defined as an attempt to counter natural desires and replace them with proscriptive rules. The desire for sweets is natural, normal, and quite pleasant! Any diet that tells you you can't have sweets, is going against your natural desire. The diet becomes a set of rigid rules, and these kinds of rules can only trigger rebellion.

Willpower does not belong in Intuitive Eating. As Marilyn became an Intuitive Eater, she found that listening to her personal signals reinforced her natural instincts, rather than fighting them. She had no one else's proscriptive rules to follow or to rebel against. Marilyn has stopped fighting the phantom willpower battle and she has lost all the weight with which she had been struggling.

Forget Being Obedient. A well-meaning suggestion by a spouse or significant other, such as: "Honey, you should have the broiled chicken ..." or "You shouldn't eat those fries ..." can set off an inner food rebellion. In this type of food combat, your only weapon to fight back becomes a double order of fries. Our clients call this *forget-you eating*.

In physics, resistance always occurs as a reaction to force. We see this principle in action in society—riots often erupt when the force of authority becomes too great. Similarly, the *simple act of being told what to do* (even if it's something you want to do) can trigger a rebellious chain reaction. Just like "terrible two-year-olds," or teenagers who revolt to prove they are independent, dieters can initiate rebellious eating in response to the act of dieting, with its set of rigid rules dictating what to eat. And so, it's not surprising to hear from our clients that breaking the rules of a diet makes them feel just like they did when they were defiant teens.

But take heart, rebellion is a normal act of self-preservation— protecting your space or personal boundaries.

Think of a personal boundary as a tall brick fence surrounding you, with only one gate. Only you can open that gate, if you choose. Therefore, no one is allowed inside, unless you invite the person in. Within your fence reside private feelings, thoughts, and biological signals. People who *assume* they know what you need and tells you what to do are picking the lock to your gate, or invading your boundaries. No one could possibly know what's inside unless you tell him, by inviting him in.

What diet or diet counselor can possibly know when you are hungry or how much food it will take to satisfy you? How can anyone but you know what texture and taste sensations will be pleasing to your palate? In the world of dieting, personal boundaries are crossed at many levels. For example, you are told what to eat, how much of it to eat, and when to eat it. These decisions should all be personal choices, with respect for individual autonomy and body signals. While food guidance may come from elsewhere, *you* should ultimately be responsible for the *when*, *what*, and *how much* of eating.

When a diet doctor or a diet plan invades your boundaries, it's normal to feel powerless. The longer you follow the food restrictions, the greater the assault to your autonomy. Here is where the paradox lies. When dieting, you will likely rebel by eating more— to restore your autonomy and protect your boundaries. But the act of rebelling can make you feel as out of control as a city riot. Instead, you have an inner food fight on your hands. But once the food rebellion is unleashed, its intensity reinforces feelings of lack of control and the belief that you don't possess willpower. Ultimately you begin to drown in a sea of self-doubt and shame. *What begins as a psychologically healthy behavior, ends in disaster.* Ultimately, weight loss is sabotaged as a result of personal boundary protection. With Intuitive Eating, there is no need to rebel, because you become the one in charge!

Boundaries are also invaded when someone makes comments about your weight or how you should look. Again, you are bound to rebel by overeating. It's a way of saying "forget you" once again; "You have no right to tell me what to weigh."

Rachel is an artist who had dieted all of her life. She was married to a successful lawyer who wanted to show off his beautiful *slim* wife to all of his colleagues. He'd continually make subtle remarks that she wasn't as thin as she could be. He would even go so far as to give her dirty looks when she reached for a rich dessert at a party. Rachel rebelled against her husband by sneaking foods behind his back (free from his evil eye). While going through the Intuitive Eating process, Rachel discovered that she was actually keeping extra weight on as the ultimate form of rebellion toward her husband.

But instead of feeling strong and powerful from her rebellion, she found that she actually felt weak, out of control, and miserable. She knew that she would feel better at her natural, lower weight, but "something" kept making her turn to the hidden extra foods. Rachel had been trapped in a game of control, boundary invasion, and rebellion all her life. Her husband and the world of dieting had been trying to control this free-spirited woman. To protect her boundaries, she would fight the diets by overeating and fight her husband's inappropriate demands by staying overweight.

Eventually, Rachel stood up to her well-meaning husband and told him that he had no right to make comments about her food or her weight. Although initially resistant, he began to respect her boundaries. She also made a firm commitment to give up dieting. As a result, Rachel was shocked to find that her secret eating disappeared, as did her self-doubt, and she began to lose weight without a struggle.

Forget About Failure. All of our chronic dieters walk into our offices feeling as if they are failures. Whether they are highly placed executives, prominent celebrities, or straight-A students, they all talk about their food experiences shamefully, and they doubt whether they'll ever be able to feel successful in the area of eating. The diet mentality reinforces feelings of success or failure. You can't fail at Intuitive Eating—it's a learning process at every point along the way. What used to be thought of as a setback, will instead be seen as a growth experience. You'll get right back on track when you see this as progress, not failure.

STEP 3:
GET RID OF THE DIETER'S TOOLS

The dieter relies on external forces to regulate his eating, sticking to a regimented food plan, eating because it's time, or eating only a specified (and measured) amount, whether hungry or not. The dieter also validates progress by external forces, primarily the scale, asking "How many pounds have I lost? Is my weight up or down?" It's time to throw out your dieting tools. Get rid of the meal plans and the bathroom scales. If all it took was a good "sensible" calorie-restricted meal plan to lose weight, we'd be a nation of thin people—free meal plans are readily available from magazines, newspapers, and even some food companies.

The Scale As False Idol. "Please, please, let the number be . . ." This wishful number prayer is not occurring in the casinos of Las Vegas, but in private homes throughout the country. But just like the desperate gambler waiting for his lucky number to come in, so is it futile for the dieter to pay homage to the "scale god." In one sweep of the scale roulette, hopes and desperation create a daily drama that will ultimately shape what mood you'll be in for the day. Ironically, "good" and "bad" scale numbers can *both* trigger overeating—whether it's a congratulatory eating celebration or a consolation party.

The scale ritual sabotages body and mind efforts; it can in one moment devalue days, weeks, and even months of progress, as illustrated with Connie.

Connie had been working very hard at Intuitive Eating and refrained from weighing herself, which in itself was a feat since she originally weighed in daily, and sometimes even twice a day at home. But Connie felt she had made so much progress in three months that she was certain she had lost a significant amount of weight. To "confirm" her progress, Connie stepped on the scale. But the number of pounds she had lost was disappointing, compared to how great she felt. The momentary brush with the scale boomeranged Connie right back to the diet mentality. That week, Connie cut back her food intake, which resulted in a large binge. Stepping on the scale was a step back into the diet mentality. It was no surprise that Connie countered her scale experience with a dieting approach. She also thought, "I must be doing something wrong." Her newfound trust began to erode—all with a single trip to the scale.

So much power is given to the almighty scale that it ultimately sabotages our efforts. But in the case of Sherry, she found the weighing process to be so humiliating that she had postponed going to doctors for fifteen years! At the age of fifty-five, Sherry had not had a mammogram or other essential physical exams because she did not want to be weighed at the doctor's office (although she weighed in at home daily). In this case, the scale was getting in the way of Sherry's health; she was at risk for breast cancer because it ran in her family. Getting the mammogram was more important than any number on the scale, but Sherry couldn't face the routine admonishments from the nursing staff. It was standard procedure—weigh the patient regardless of the reason for the appointment. Sherry did not realize that she had the right to refuse to be weighed. She finally got the courage after our work together. She made a doctor's appointment and refused to be weighed since it was not an essential component of her medical care at the moment. Fortunately her physical exam results were healthy.

We have found that the "weigh-in" factor usually detracts from a person's progress. In the "old days" when we used to weigh all patients, we found that sessions were often spent on why the weight went up or did not move at all, and they became scale-counseling sessions. Our patients also dreaded the weighing-in part as much as we did.

When a Pound Is Not a Pound. Many factors can influence a person's weight which do *not* reflect that person's body fat. For example, two cups of water weigh one pound. If you tend to retain water or bloat, the scale can easily rise a few pounds without a change in what you have eaten. But for the oft guilt-ridden dieter, the consequences of water weight can seem severe. For example, we have had many patients feel bad about eating an extra dessert over the weekend and weigh themselves on the following Monday. The scale shoots up five pounds—and they *believe* they gained five pounds of *fat*. Since many dieter-clients are quick with the calorie calculator, we ask, "Did you eat an *extra* 17,500 calories over the weekend?" Of course not, would be their retort. Yet to make five pounds of fat requires a caloric *excess* of 17,500 calories above normal eating (one pound of fat is equivalent to 3,500 calories).

So how do you explain the weight gain? Water weight. Any time the scale suddenly rises or falls, it is usually because of a fluid shift in the body. Eating high-sodium foods can also provoke water retention (not fat retention) in salt-sensitive individuals. Yet how easily chronic dieters believe they did something wrong; they must have single-handedly gobbled five pounds worth of food! No! No! No!

Similarly, losing two pounds immediately from an hour of aerobics is not a two-pound fat loss. Rather, it's mostly water loss from sweat.

Jubilant dieters who think that they have lost ten pounds in a week may be in for an unwanted surprise. While it may be true that the scale indicated ten pounds less than when they weighed one week ago, the question is, what *kind* of weight did they lose? To lose ten pounds of fat in one week requires an energy deficit of 35,000 calories, or a deficit of 5,000 calories each day! The average woman only eats about 1,500 to 1,600 calories per day. The sad reality is that this person is losing a lot of water weight, usually at the expense of their muscles, due to the process of *muscle-wasting*. Muscle is made up mainly of water (about 70 percent).

When a hungry body is not given enough calories, the body cannibalizes itself for an energy source. The prime directive of the body is that it must have energy, at any cost—it's part of the survival mechanism. The protein in muscles is converted to valuable energy for the body. When a muscle cell is destroyed, water is released and eventually excreted—there's your precious weight loss. The whittled-away muscle contributes to lowering your metabolism. Muscles are metabolically active tissue—generally the more muscle we have, the higher our metabolic rate. That's one of the reasons men burn more calories than women—they have more muscle mass.

Increased muscle mass, while metabolically more active and desirable, weighs more than fat. Muscle also takes up less space than fat. While this is certainly beneficial, a chronic dieter often gets frustrated by the rising, or unchanging, scale number. *The scale does*

Issue	Diet Mentality	Nondiet Mentality
SUMMARY: THE DIET MENTALITY VERSUS THE NONDIET MENTALITY		
Eating/Food Choices	•Do I deserve it? •If I eat a heavy food, I try to find a way to make up for it. •I feel guilty when I eat heavy foods. •I usually describe a day of eating as either good or bad. •I view food as the enemy.	•Am I hungry? •Do I want it? •Will I be deprived if I don't eat it? •Will it be satisfying? •Does it taste good? •I deserve to enjoy eating without guilt.
Exercise Benefits	•I focus primarily on the calories burned. •I feel guilty if I miss a designated exercise day.	•I focus primarily on how exercise makes me feel, especially the energizing and stress-relieving factors.
View of Progress	•How many pounds did I lose? •How do I look? •What do other people think of my weight? •I have good willpower.	•While I'm concerned with my weight, it is not my primary goal or indicator of progress. •I have increased trust with myself and food. •I am able to let go of "eating indiscretions." •I recognize inner body cues.

not reflect body composition—just like weighing a piece of steak at the butcher's does not tell you how lean the meat is.

Weighing in on the scale only serves to keep you focused on your weight; it doesn't help with the process of getting back in touch with Intuitive Eating. Constant weigh-ins can leave you frustrated and impede your progress. Best bet—stop weighing yourself.

INTUITIVE EATING TOOLS

The tools of the Intuitive Eater are internal cues, not outside forces telling you what, when, and how much to eat. But to acquire and understand these internal cues, you need a new set of power tools— or rather, *em*power*ment* tools, which will be discussed in the following chapters.

Chapter Six

Honor Your Hunger

Keep your body fed biologically with adequate energy and carbohydrates. Otherwise, you can trigger a primal drive to overeat. Once you reach the moment of excessive hunger, all intentions of moderate, conscious eating are fleeting and irrelevant. Learning to honor this first biological signal sets the stage for rebuilding trust with yourself and food.

A dieting body is a starving body. Drastic comparison? No. While a dieting body may not *look* like a starving person in Ethiopia or Somalia, the "symptoms" from dieting exhibit a striking resemblance to the starvation state. The body does not know that there is a McDonald's on every corner as you embark on a diet. As far as the body is concerned, it is living in a famine state and needs to adapt. Our need for food (energy) is so essential and primal that if we are not getting enough energy, our bodies naturally compensate with powerful biological and psychological mechanisms.

The power of food deprivation was keenly demonstrated in a landmark starvation study conducted by Dr. Ancel Keys during World War II, designed to help famine sufferers. The subjects of the study were thirty-two healthy men who were selected because they had superior "psychobiological stamina"—superior mental and physical health.

During the first three months of the study the men ate as they pleased, averaging 3,492 calories per day. The next six months was the semistarvation period. The men were required to lose 19 to 28 percent of their weight depending on their body composition.

Calories were cut nearly in half, to an average of 1,570 per day. The effects of the semistarvation were startling, and strikingly mirror the symptoms of chronic dieting:

- Metabolic rates decreased by 40 percent.

- The men were obsessed with food. They had heightened food cravings and talked of food and collecting recipes.

- Eating style changed—vacillating from ravenous gulping to stalling out the eating experience. Some men played with their food and dawdled over a meal for two hours.

- The researchers noted that, "Several men failed to adhere to their diets and reported episodes of bulimia." One man was reported to have suffered a complete loss of "willpower" and ate several cookies, a sack of popcorn, and two bananas. Another subject "flagrantly broke the dietary rules" and ate several sundaes and malted milks, and even stole penny candy.

- Some men exercised deliberately to obtain increased food rations.

- Personalities changed, and in many cases there was the onset of apathy, irritability, moodiness and depression.

During the refeeding period when the men were once again allowed to eat at will, hunger became insatiable. The men found it difficult to stop eating. Weekend splurges added up to 8,000 to 10,000 calories. It took the majority of men an average of five months to normalize their eating.

It's important to remember that during the era of this classic study, there were no Arnold Schwarzeneggers or fitness and food divas. Nutrition research was just in its infancy. Yet these men experienced a primal obsession with food that was not media-driven or society-driven; rather it was triggered by a biological survival mechanism. Such behavior had never been observed in these men prior to their food-deprivation encounter! Although this is a classic starvation study, the caloric level is representative of a modern weight-loss diet for men of 1,500 calories. These men were eating. Imagine if the same study was held under today's pressures to be thin.

We have had several clients read the classic Keys study and they are struck by the similarity of their own experiences to those of the semistarved men. Mary, for example, noted that after completing her second liquid fast program she was more obsessed with food than ever before. She bought several cookbooks and major cooking appliances—a waffle maker, a bread maker, and a food processor. The biggest paradox Mary noted was that she doesn't like to cook and did not use her new appliances or cookbooks!

Jan had dieted most of her life. But the more she dieted the more interested she got in food. She collected magazine and newspaper recipes of all kinds, from rich gourmet to spartan spa cuisine, and read them as if they were engaging novels. Yet she would never dare prepare the scrumptious recipes; instead, they were her food fantasies and food escapism.

Of Mice and Men. Rats are certainly not exposed to the social pressures and nuances of eating that humans are, yet when deprived of food, rats will also overeat. In one study, rats were divided into two groups, one food-deprived and one control group. The food-deprived rats went without food for up to four days, and then were allowed to eat again until they gained their weight back. Both groups of rats were then given free access to a "palatable diet"—beyond the ordinary rat chow staples, like five-star dining in the rodent world. While both groups gained weight, those in the food-deprived group gained more weight, *in direct proportion to the length of their prior deprivation.*

PRIMAL HUNGER

The psychological terror of hunger is profound, notes Naomi Wolf in her book, *The Beauty Myth*. Even after hunger has ended, the nagging terror of it remains. She cites how hungry orphans adopted from poor countries often cannot control their compulsion to smuggle and hide food, even after living for years in a secure environment. A disproportionate number of concentration camp survivors are now obese.

Research historians have documented that during times of famine or food shortages, food becomes an overriding preoccupation resulting in societal problems: breakdown of social behavior, abandonment of cooperative effort, loss of personal pride and sense of family ties. While this preoccupation with food has been observed during times of food deprivation, these actions also mirror dieting behavior at the individual level. How often have you become more socially isolated while on a diet, turning down a party invitation, for instance, because you didn't want to deal with the food, or not going out altogether until you are through with your diet?

While the hunger and food obsession from dieting may not be experienced as a terrifying event, it does leave a lasting mark.

Karen had been on several medically supervised fasts over her lifetime and became frightened of experiencing hunger. To her, hunger *was* terrifying and often resulted in out-of-control eating which reinforced her fear of hunger. Therefore, Karen always kept herself in a "fed" state between diets, and never really experienced gentle biological hunger. She only knew what *extreme* hunger felt like, with all of its voracious intensity. To avoid hunger she was constantly eating, but the persistent eating caused more weight gain, so she would start a new diet or fasting program and the vicious cycle would continue—hunger from dieting, followed by overeating.

MECHANISMS THAT TRIGGER EATING

Whether or not you are a chronic dieter, powerful biological mechanisms are triggered when your body does not get the energy from food that it needs. It's no accident that food is included as one of the fundamental human needs in Maslow's Hierarchy of Needs—a model that ranks human needs, suggesting that certain basic needs must be met before you can go on to fulfill more complex ones. Food and energy are so essential to the survival of the human species that if we don't eat enough we set off a biological fuse that turns on our eating drive both physically and psychologically. The hunger drive is truly a mind-body connection. Eating is so important that the nerve cells of appetite are located in the hypothalamus region of the brain. A variety of biological signals trigger eating. What many people believe to be an issue of willpower is instead a *biological drive.* The power and intensity of the biological eating drive should not be underestimated. The neurochemicals from the brain coordinate our eating behavior with our body's biological need. Through a complex system of chemical and neural feedback, the brain monitors the energy needs of all our body systems, moment to moment. And it makes very emphatic chemical directives as to what we should eat. Fasting or restricting is particularly detrimental to appetite control. It simply turns on the neurochemical switches that induce us to eat.

Many studies have shown that lowering body weight by food restriction and dieting makes no sense metabolically or to our brain chemistry. In fact, it's counterproductive. The biological chemicals that regulate appetite also directly affect moods and state of mind, our physical energy and our sex lives.

Most researchers agree that there are both complex biological *and* psychological mechanisms that influence our eating. In this chapter we will focus on the profound biological mechanisms that turn on our desire to eat, especially if we have been food-deprived or dieting.

Heightened Digestion

In food-deprived individuals, research has shown that the body gets biologically primed for the moment of eating, like a sprinter crouched in a ready-position for an explosive start, the moment the starting pistol is triggered.

- Salivation increases with increases of food deprivation, even when there is no food present or suggestion of eating! This has been demonstrated in studies both on dieters and normal (nondieting) individuals.

- Increased digestive hormones have been found in dieters both before and after eating.

The Carbohydrate Craver: Neuropeptide Y

Neuropeptide Y (NPY) is a chemical produced by the brain that triggers our drive to eat carbohydrates, the body's primary and preferred source of energy. While most of what we know about NPY comes from research on rats, there is a lot of evidence that shows that this brain chemical can have a profound impact on human eating behavior as well by increasing both the size and duration of carbohydrate-rich meals.

Food deprivation or undereating drives NPY into action, causing the body to seek more carbohydrates. When the next meal or eating opportunity rolls around, it can easily turn into a high-carbohydrate binge—not because you lack willpower or are out of control; it's your biology (rather, NPY) screaming, "Feed me."

NPY is revved up after any imposed period of food deprivation, including an overnight fast from dinner to breakfast. NPY's levels are naturally the highest in the morning because of the short-term food deprivation from an overnight fast. The elevated NPY levels are part of the biological basis for eating in the morning! During an overnight fast, your body's stores of carbohydrates in the liver are drained and need refilling. You literally wake up on empty in the morning. But if you skip breakfast, you are likely to pay for it with increases in NPY level, which can lead into mid-afternoon gorging.

The brain also makes more NPY when carbohydrates are being burned as fuel and in times of stress. Eating carbohydrates turns off NPY through its effect on serotonin, another brain chemical. As we eat more carbohydrates, it helps to increase the production of serotonin, which in turn shuts off the production of NPY and puts a halt to the desire for carbohydrates.

The more you deny your true hunger and fight your natural biology, the stronger and more intense food cravings and obsessions become. Fasting or restricting especially revs up the NPY and drives the body to seek more carbohydrates. So by the time the next eating opportunity occurs, it can *easily* become a high-carbohydrate binge.

Why is there such a chemical drive for carbohydrates? Let's look briefly at the critical role carbohydrates play in the body—it will help you understand the primal hunger drive.

The Importance of Carbohydrates. Carbohydrates are the gold standard of food energy to the body. Cells function best when they receive a certain level of carbohydrates, in the form of glucose, and even small decreases can cause problems. The brain, nervous system, and red blood cells rely *exclusively* on glucose for fuel. Because of the importance of glucose, the levels of it in the blood are closely regulated by two hormones, insulin and glucagon.

There is a very limited amount of carbohydrate stored in the liver, in the form of glycogen, that helps supply more glucose to the blood when levels get too low. Yet this precious fuel reserve ordinarily lasts only three to six hours (except at night, when liver glycogen lasts longer because the need for energy is lower). How does this fuel reserve get replaced? Eating. Eating carbohydrate-rich foods, that is.

If a diet is lacking in carbohydrates, the body has to turn to creative fueling mechanisms to supply vital energy to the body. Protein mainly from muscle will get taken apart and converted to energy, primarily in the form of glucose. It's like taking wood from the framework structure in your house to use as fuel in your fireplace. The wood will burn and provide necessary fuel, but it does so at a high price. You begin to lose the integrity of your structure!

If you think that eating a high-protein diet will prevent this dismantling from occurring, it's not so. When you eat an inadequate amount of energy, or carbohydrates, the protein from the diet will *also* be diverted to be used as energy. Therefore this "high-protein diet" is no insurance. Instead, the protein is used as an expensive source of fuel, rather than for its intended use in the body. It's like having a building supplier provide lots of wood to rebuild your house. If you are constantly using that wood pile to make bonfires instead of to repair your home, you are still left with a weak structure. Similarly, protein is needed to maintain and build muscles, hormones, enzymes, and cells in the body. When carbohydrates and energy are lacking, protein is shifted from its primary role to provide fuel.

Many of our clients believe that when we don't have enough energy, our bodies will finally start burning fat. It doesn't work that way. Remember, the brain and other parts of the body need carbohydrates exclusively for fuel. Only a very small component (5 percent) of the stored fat can be converted to a carbohydrate fuel. On the other hand, the body has plenty of enzymes to convert protein to glucose.

One reason people lose weight so quickly on low-carbohydrate or fasting diets is that they are devouring their own protein tissues as fuel. Since protein contains only half as many calories per pound as fat, it disappears twice as fast. With each pound of body protein, three or four pounds of associated water are lost. If your body were to continue to consume itself at this rate, death would occur within about ten days. After all, the liver, heart muscle, and lung tissue— all vital tissues—are being burned as fuel. Even when the heart muscle is deteriorating, it still has to keep up the same amount of work, with *less* power and at a slower heart rate. In essence, the cannibalized heart muscle has to work harder with a smaller, faulty engine; pumping performance is not reduced in proportion to the amount of heart tissue lost.

Eventually, the body can convert stored fat to a form of usable energy for the brain and nervous system called ketones. This process is known as ketosis. Ketosis is an adaptation to prolonged fasting or carbohydrate deprivation. But only about *half* of the brain's cells can use these compounds for energy. Therefore, when fat is being used under these deprivation conditions, the body's lean tissue (protein) continues to be lost at a rapid rate in order to supply glucose to nervous system cells that cannot use ketones as fuel. The bottom line? Adequate carbohydrates and energy are important!

The Powerhouse Cell Theory

Hunger signals are not affected by low carbohydrates alone. According to the work of cellular researchers Nicolaidis and Even, the hunger signal is generated by the overall energy need of the cell. When cellular power is low, it will produce a signal that induces hunger. While cells get their energy primarily from carbohydrate, protein and fat are factored into the cellular power equation, which could trigger hunger. For example, even if one of your household appliances runs on pure electricity, it could also get its energy from batteries, or a gasoline-powered generator. They all provide energy, but have different costs and efficiencies. All nutrients that provide energy (carbohydrates, protein, and fat) eventually get converted to one universal energy denomination used by the cells, ATP. ATP is the chemical energy that powers the cells, and thus our bodies.

Nicolaidis and Even propose that the hunger signal is triggered by the overall ATP need of the cell.

To sum up—we need energy. Energy comes from food.

Second-Guessing Your Biology

In spite of the complex and elegant biological systems that help ensure our bodies get enough energy (food), all too often the chronic dieter tries to outthink biology. Rather than eating when hungry, eating is often tied into a cognitive set point, based on the dieter's set of rules (Is it time? Do I deserve it? Is it too much? And so forth). For example, on the days Alice exercised, early in the morning, she would get mad at herself for eating a larger (but appropriate) breakfast. She was worried that her body did not deserve the "extra" portion of food, so her solution was to skip lunch. Skipping lunch was easy, because Alice was a busy executive assistant, with never enough hours in the day to get her work done. Her busyness preoccupied any afternoon hunger that would surface. But by the time Alice arrived at home in the evening, she would be so hungry she would overeat at dinner and often late into the night. Or if she was eating out at a restaurant she would devour the bread basket and clean her plate, feeling stuffed and guilty by the end of her meal.

Even nondieters who go too long without eating will often overeat. (Remember, even rats overeat when food-deprived.) You are also likely to buy more food impulsively when you are in a ravenous state, regardless of your health and dieting intentions.

The problem with consistently denying your hunger state is twofold. First, it usually crescendos into a period of overeating. Secondly, when the mind gets so used to ignoring hunger signals, they begin to fade and you don't hear them anymore. Or you can only "hear" hunger in extreme, ravenous states, which can be adverse. This further conditions you to believe that you can't be trusted with food, because ravenous hunger often triggers overeating. This is explained in part by the Boundary Model for the Regulation of Eating developed by C. Peter Herman and Janet Polivy, psychological experts in chronic dieting. This model considers both the biology and psychology of eating.

The Boundary model explains how dieters, through their cognitive set point, push their normal biological cues of hunger and satiety to the extremes. The gentle sensations of hunger are atrophied for a dieter who is constantly trying to suppress them. Instead, the dieter might only feel extreme, ravenous hunger—or be so disconnected that the feeling of hunger is difficult to identify. Similarly, for this individual, it can be increasingly difficult to know what comfortable satiety feels like. Instead, the dieter hovers in a gray zone of what Herman and Polivy call "biological indifference." In the zone of biological indifference, there is no clear hunger or satiety cue. This zone is so wide for the chronic dieter that instead of eating based on internal eating cues—food thoughts and judgments prevail and tell the dieter what to do.

PRIMAL FOOD THERAPY:
HONOR YOUR HUNGER

The first step to reclaiming the world of normal eating, free of dieting and food worry, is to *honor your biological hunger*. Your body needs to *know* consistently that it will have access to food—that dieting and deprivation have halted, once and for all. Otherwise, your biology will always be on call, ready to avert a self-imposed food deprivation.

Your body needs to be biologically reconditioned. Diet after diet has taught your body that personal famines are frequent, so it should stay on guard. Remember, famines and food shortages have always existed, even in our modern times. Our bodies are still biologically equipped to survive famines through lowering our energy requirements, increasing biological chemicals that trigger our eating drive, and so on.

It is much easier to stop eating when your body isn't starving. For example, imagine you are in a room and offer a *starving* child a plate of cookies. You tell the child that she can have only one cookie. You exit the room and leave the child alone with the whole plate. What would the hungry child do? Eat all the cookies (and lick the crumbs), of course. But if the child knew that cookies (or any other food) were always available when hungry, the intense drive to eat would be greatly diminished. The same is true for dieters.

For example, Barbara usually kept herself in a hungry state. She only allowed herself to eat when extremely ravenous. By her own definition, if she allowed herself to eat when simply hungry, *but not ravenous*, she thought she was overeating. Yet because her definition of "normal" hunger was being ravenous, her eating would vacillate from feast to famine cycles.

HUNGER SILENCE

What if you don't feel hunger anymore, or don't really know what the gentle sensation of hunger feels like? Can you get it back? Yes. But first let's look at a couple of reasons why hunger may be silenced.

• *Numbing.* Many people have learned over the years to quell, or avert hunger pangs by turning to calorie-free beverages, such as diet sodas, coffee, and tea. The liquid in the stomach temporarily tricks the gastric mechanism into a sense of fullness.

• *Dieting.* Dieters get so used to denying their hunger that it becomes easy to tune it out. Eventually, when hunger comes knocking on their inner door and there is no response, the knocking, or rather the stomach rumbling, stops.

• *Chaos.* It's very easy to suppress hunger or ignore it, when you are busy putting out the fires in your life or job. If this is a chronic pattern, hunger may slowly fade.

• *Skipping Breakfast.* Some of our clients skip breakfast in the morning, because they say it keeps them feeling hungrier the rest of the day or because they're in a hurry. Yet hunger is a normal, welcomed body signal that should be embraced. It's a sign that you are getting back in touch with your body's needs. But because these clients are afraid of their hunger, they respond by not eating breakfast the next morning—which repeats the vicious cycle of hunger silence.

HOW TO HONOR BIOLOGICAL HUNGER

It's too hard to hear hunger if you are never listening for it. The first step to honoring your biological hunger is to begin to listen for it. The symphony of hunger has many sounds that are varied for different people. Just as an orchestra conductor can distinguish the voices of each instrument in a symphony you will eventually be able to key in to specific bodily sensations and what they mean. In the beginning, you may be able to recognize overt ravenous hunger, but have difficulty recognizing gentle hunger pangs. Similarly, to the nontrained musical ear, loud cymbals might be easy to identify, but it will take time and listening to pick up on the subtler voices of the bassoon or oboe.

Each time you eat, ask yourself: "Am I hungry? What's my hunger level?" If the feeling of hunger is hard to identify, ask yourself: "When was the last time I *ever* felt hungry? How did my stomach feel? How did my mouth feel?" Any combination of the following can be experienced as hunger sensations or symptoms (ranging from gentle to ravenous):

- Mild gurgling or gnawing in the stomach
- Growling noises
- Light-headedness
- Difficulty concentrating
- Uncomfortable stomach pain
- Irritability
- Feeling faint
- Headache

The ebb and flow of your hunger might not match other people's—that's okay, it's individual. Take care not to get overly hungry or ravenous. If this is difficult for you to gauge, a general guideline is to *go no longer than five waking hours without eating.* This is based on the biology of fueling up your carbohydrate tank in the liver, which runs out every three to six hours. We have observed that clients who go longer than five hours without eating tend to overeat at the next eating opportunity.

To get in touch with the nuances of hunger, it helps to check the pulse of hunger at regular intervals. Check in with your body, and simply inquire, What's my hunger level? It's helpful to do this every time you eat, and between eating occurrences. Remember, although this may seem hyperconscious, it's a focused step to get you reacquainted with your body and its biology.

We have used a variety of tools to help our clients check in with their hunger, but one is particularly helpful and is a little less exacting. Monitor your hunger level each time you eat, before and after, using the Hunger Discovery Scale. What pattern do you see emerging? Is there a certain time interval when you eat? Is there any relationship between how much you eat and the length of time between eating?

You may discover that your eating style leans toward nibbling or grazing. Don't be alarmed. If you eat small amounts of food such as a snack or mini-meal, you may find that you are hungry more often, such as every three to four hours. Not only is this normal, it may have metabolic advantages. Nibbling studies (in which people are given multiple snacks or mini-meals) have shown that the release of insulin is lower in people fed nibbling diets compared to larger traditional meals of *identical* calories. Insulin is a fat-building hormone. The more insulin released, the easier it is for the body to make fat.

Sometimes our clients get worried when they suddenly feel more hungry than usual—as if something is wrong. However, on closer inspection, they usually find that a couple of days prior they had an unusually light day of eating—not dieting, but just not a lot of food. The body plays catch-up on its own terms. Most of our clients have difficulty remembering what they ate one day ago, let alone two days ago. Research on children has shown that they make up for their nutritional needs in an average of time from a couple of days to a week. Why should adults be any different? In fact, new research is beginning to indicate the same *is* true for adults. The body may do some of its energy fine-tuning over a period of days, rather than from hour to hour. We find this is especially true if you still have a tendency to eat diet types of food such as rice cakes or salad. You may feel full, but the lack of energy catches up with you. The body wants to compensate.

Other Voices of "Hunger"

A common mistake with our newer clients is that they initially embrace the *honor your hunger* concept in the form of a diet mantra, "Thou shall eat only when hungry." The problem here is that this rigid interpretation can leave you feeling as if you have broken a

THE HUNGER DISCOVERY SCALE

Time	Food	Hunger Rating										
		0	1	2	3	4	5	6	7	8	9	10

Empty   Set   **Neutral**   Full   Sick

Ravenous   Pangs   Satisfied   Stuffed

◄   0   1   2   3   4   5   6   7   8   9   10   ►

Use this scale (0–10) to help you identify your initial hunger when you begin to eat. This rating system is purely subjective and will help you get in touch with your body's inner signals. The neutral point is 5, when you are neither hungry nor full. Visualize your stomach getting emptier and hungrier as you go down on the scale to a 0, completely empty. At 4, you begin to feel the first awakening of hunger. Hunger pangs begin there and increase to a 3. By 2, your hunger is completely set, and you're feeling quite hungry. At 1, you are ravenous.

Every time you start to eat, check your hunger level. Ideally it should be at a 3 or 4 level. If you are at a 5 or above, you're not biologically hungry. If you're at 2 or lower, you're overhungry and at risk for overeating.

rule, or failed, if you eat for any other reason than hunger. When you feel like you have broken a rule, you can get pulled right back into the diet mentality. It's important to recognize that normal eaters don't always eat just from pure hunger, yet they maintain their weight.

- *Taste Hunger.* Sometimes people may eat simply because it sounds good or because the occasion calls for it. We call this *taste hunger.* Normal eaters can accept this—they don't view it as a big diet violation. In nearly every culture, food plays an important role in rites of passages and celebratory events. Would you chastise a bride or groom for eating a piece of wedding cake when she or he was not hungry? Yet it's not unusual for dieters to feel bad about *any* perceived food transgression, and then feel like they might as well throw in the towel. And that's when overeating often takes place.

- *Practical "Hunger"—Planning Ahead.* While it's important to eat primarily based on your biological hunger, it's also important to be practical and not rigid. For instance, let's say you are attending a play with friends that lasts from 7:00 to 10:00 P.M. and your opportunity to eat is at 6:00 P.M. You may not be hungry then, but you certainly will be later. Do you sit there at the restaurant and *not* eat, and let hunger roll in right in the middle of the play, only to culminate in ravenous hunger by the final act? No. Eating a light meal or snack beforehand is a sensible solution.

- *Emotional Hunger.* Once you are truly able to identify and distinguish biological hunger, it becomes easier to clarify *why* you want to eat. It is not unusual for a number of our clients to eat because of *emotional hunger*—to quench uncomfortable feelings (such as loneliness, boredom, and anger). Ironically, many of our clients are often amazed that what they assumed to be emotional eating was in many instances primal-hunger eating. But the out-of-control feeling of overeating is nearly identical, whether it was triggered emotionally or biologically. A discussion of how to distinguish the sources of hunger is found in Chapter 11.

Chapter Seven

PRINCIPLE 3:

Make Peace with Food

Call a truce; stop the food fight! Give yourself unconditional permission to eat. If you tell yourself that you can't or shouldn't have a particular food, it can lead to intense feelings of deprivation that build into uncontrollable cravings and, often, bingeing. When you finally "give in" to your forbidden foods, eating will be experienced with such intensity, it usually results in Last Supper overeating and overwhelming guilt.

When I was on the Grapefruit Diet, all I wanted was bananas, and when I was on a low-carbohydrate diet, all I did was dream of eating bread and potatoes," said Laurie, an inveterate dieter. Does that sound ironic? Familiar? What may seem like irony is actually the natural reaction that is triggered by the limitation and deprivation that comes with most diets.

Cravings run rampant as soon as we're restricted from any kind of substance—whether it is clothing, fresh air, scenery, or especially food. Scientists living in the Biosphere 2, an experimental airtight glass-enclosed terrarium, coveted something as basic as fresh air after being deprived of an open environment for two years. But fresh air was not the only fantasy of these researchers—so was the food they had sorely missed. After they emerged from this self-imposed captivity, the research team had more to say about food than science at their press conference. The scientists described cravings for food that began to occupy their thoughts and led one of them to write a cookbook!

These scientists are not unlike the dieter who has been told certain foods are forbidden. Even though they were not on a diet, the scientists were still preoccupied with food cravings as a result of lack of availability. They dreamed about desserts which were nonexistent and obsessed about dinners, which were of limited variety. As cooking chores rotated, it became vitally important not to spoil the day's meal for the others. Common foods like salmon, berries, and coffee took on a heightened allure.

THE DEPRIVATION SET-UP

Why would Biosphere scientists or the healthy men in the Ancel Keys study (described in the previous chapter) exhibit behaviors so unlike their normal eating patterns? Deprivation. These people had not been tainted by the dieting trap, yet their reactions to deprivation were virtually identical to those of dieters. While you have already seen the effects of *biological* deprivation in the last chapter, you should not underestimate the effect of deprivation *psychologically*. This effect is the focus of this chapter.

When you rigidly limit the amount of food you are allowed to eat, it usually sets you up to crave *larger* quantities of that very food. In fact, being restricted from anything in life sets it up to be extra special, regardless of age. (Oh, maybe not in the beginning, when you are in the initial stages of diet euphoria, but the craving builds with each "dieting day.") For example, if you put a two-year-old on the floor with several brand-new toys and tell him that he can play with any one of them except for the simple oatmeal carton, which do you think he'll choose? You guessed it—the plain oatmeal carton.

One client revealed that when he was young, he had little money and the thought of buying a new car gave him a deep thrill. Yet, now that he's successful and can buy *any* car he wants at any time, cars are no longer a big deal, no thrill. Food has replaced the thrill that buying a new car used to provide. Paradoxically, food is the one thing out of his reach, forbidden, when dieting. The forbidden object is elevated to an overvalued level of specialness.

Psychologist Fritz Heider states that depriving yourself of something you want can actually heighten your desire for that very item. *The moment you banish a food, it paradoxically builds up a "craving life" of its own that gets stronger with each diet, and builds more momentum as the deprivation deepens.* Deprivation is a powerful experience both biologically and psychologically. You saw in the last chapter how food deprivation sets off a biological drive. Psychological forces wreak havoc with your peace of mind, triggering cravings, obsessive thoughts, and even compulsive behaviors. If you are someone who has also experienced deprivation in areas outside of food, such as love, attention, material wants, etc., the deprivation connected to dieting may be felt even more intensely for you. Bonnie is a client who grew up in a home where her father was never home and her mother was emotionally distant. As a young child, she learned to use food as a way to substitute for the love and attention she wasn't getting. As an adult on a diet, she found that food deprivation evoked these deep feelings of deprivation from childhood. For Bonnie, this became a double whammy which was hard to overcome. For the chronic dieter, the combination of biological changes (from undereating), psychological reactions, and cognitive distortions create just the right mix to set off the dynamite of rebound eating.

DEPRIVATION BACKLASH— ## REBOUND EATING

Meet Heidi. Her experience with chocolate typifies what can happen when you deprive yourself of a particular food. Heidi had been on every known diet, each forbidding one type of food or another, and chocolate was almost always on the "do not eat" list. Heidi was a self-described chocoholic. She complained that the moment chocolate crossed her lips, she couldn't stop eating it. Her way of managing her chocolate problem was simply to not allow herself to eat it. But this was a vicious cycle. It was not uncommon for Heidi to consume large boxes of chocolate in spite of her attempts to eliminate it from her life. The moment a box of chocolate was opened, she couldn't resist eating it to completion. Heidi's chocolate binges were triggered by the food rule she had created—"I am not allowed to eat chocolate." This meant that each time she "succumbed" and ate it, she truly believed that it was for the last time. Each chocolate episode would become a "farewell to chocolate," with all the sadness and mourning that goes along with saying good-bye to anything special in life. Since Heidi "knew" she was never, *ever* going to eat chocolate again (despite her experience demonstrating otherwise), she would consume large amounts of it as a last hurrah, or "get it while you can." When Heidi's chocolate binges occurred, she would feel guilty and as if she did not deserve to eat any food. She would compensate for her chocolate feasts by undereating or semi-fasting, which would set her up for ravenous hunger and more out-of-control eating.

Today, Heidi eats chocolate but is often satisfied with a piece or two, and can easily even pass it up! To Heidi, this is a miracle. How did she overcome her chocolate problem? Heidi's solution was to learn to make peace with food—especially with chocolate—an idea that she was terrified to try in the beginning. No wonder; her only experience with chocolate was eating it in massive quantities, then feeling out of control. For Heidi, making peace with chocolate was a brave and risky step.

Last Supper Eating

The mere perception that food might become banned can trigger overeating. Just thinking about going on a diet can create a sense of panic and send you on a trail of eating every food that you think won't be allowed. As we explained in Chapter 1, this is Last Supper eating. It is triggered by the sincere belief that you will never get to eat a particular food (or foods) again. The threat of deprivation becomes so powerful that all reason is lost and you find yourself eating whatever is to be forbidden, even if you are not hungry.

Clients will often overeat right before their first session. Although we make it clear that we use a nondieting approach, they figure that we have something up our sleeves, a diet of sorts—after all, we are nutritionists! For example, Paul ate in an out-of-control fashion the night before his first appointment. Why? Paul was sure that he would be advised to give up most of his favorite foods and start eating a diet of carrots and cottage cheese. His fear increased during the week leading up to his session, and so did his intake of french fries, hamburgers, and donuts. This experience was not new to Paul—in fact, he had engaged in Last Supper eating before *every* diet he started. Likewise, nearly all of our clients engage in this predieting ritual of saying good-bye to favorite foods. In fact, some of our clients tell us that Last Supper eating is one of their favorite parts of dieting—it's almost an entitlement.

For some of our clients, however, there is such an intense sense of urgency with Last Supper eating that a period of frantic gorging ensues. One client described it as, "Hurry and get all the food while you can, and time is short, so get it all, now!" The overeating that follows falsely gives "proof" that you need to diet, as you watch in horror your inability to "control" yourself.

Each impending diet brings with it more fear of deprivation—with the knowledge that you won't get "enough" or get what you want. Then comes more overeating, loss of self-control, and, finally, erosion of self-esteem. How could you possibly feel good about yourself if you truly believe that it's possible to eliminate certain foods, only to find yourself bingeing and failing on yet another diet?

Rebound Eating: Subtle Forms

Food Competition. Have you ever shared a bowl of cherries or a piece of dessert with someone who eats faster than you? Watch how quickly you dig in because you're concerned that you won't get enough. Or see what happens when you hear that your favorite brand of cereal is to be discontinued; it's not unusual to buy every last box on the shelf because of fear of deprivation. Or some parents find themselves gobbling down the cookies before the kids can get their hands on them.

Eating in a large group of people can instill a sense of future food-deprivation worry. To prevent this from occurring, there is a tendency to eat quickly, grab it while you can, or there won't be any food left. For example, Joshua was one of nine children in a family of moderate means. As a child he was worried that he wouldn't get enough food at mealtime, although in actuality there was an adequate amount of food to go around. While not overweight as a child, the fear of food deprivation taught him to grab what he could. As an adult he continued this behavior, which evolved into an obesity problem.

Returning Home Syndrome. When they return from having been away, people often overeat because they felt deprived of familiar foods while away. Kids returning home from summer camp or from their college dorms find themselves emptying the refrigerator, gorging on home cooking, or visiting their favorite local restaurants excessively. Recently, I (ER) came home to find my stepson's friend, who had just returned from Thailand, methodically eating everything in the kitchen that he hadn't seen in three years. When he began to eat the cream cheese by the forkful (without a bagel), I knew how deprived he had been! Even fresh fruits and vegetables take on a heightened allure when one is returning from a journey in which they were not available. For example, clients have described unusual cravings for salads after a two-week camping trip or a trip abroad where it's been advised *not* to eat the fresh produce.

The Empty Cupboard. If there is consistently no food in the house because grocery shopping is chaotic, eating often vacillates between feast and famine, with emphasis on the former. Food in the pantry or refrigerator takes on extra specialness.

For example, Gayle is a young woman who exhibits a tendency to eat every bite of food in a meal regardless of how stuffed she feels. Gayle's parents work many hours, seldom shop for food, and eat most of their meals out. Gayle usually comes home from school to an empty house, no food or parents. With food haphazardly available, Gayle feels greatly deprived. She feels a compulsion to finish whatever food she gets, as she doesn't know where or when her next meal will appear.

Captivity Behavior. Accounts of released hostages have reported obsessive thinking about food and cravings while "in captivity." On a somewhat lighter level, my (ER) son described his "captivity" behavior during a survival training camp out in the wilderness in Montana. To occupy his lonely hours, he would write lists of all the foods he wasn't getting. Yet normally, he is not preoccupied with food or cravings.

Depression Era Eating. People who went through the Great American Depression hold food in special regard; it's cherished. There is a pervasive sense that there won't be enough food, or certain foods may become unavailable. And like a precious metal, you dare not throw food away, let alone waste it. "Clean your plate" takes on special meaning, and is passed on with other family traditions and values.

Once in a Lifetime. Eating a meal in a special restaurant while on vacation can stimulate a sense of future deprivation. For example, if you are in Paris eating a superb French meal, the thought of leaving even a forkful seems an impossible feat. After all, this is likely to be the one and only time you'll ever experience these particular tastes in this particular setting! You might eat until you're uncomfortably full, just because you're already feeling deprived.

One Last Shot. A similar experience can occur when eating a delicious meal at the home of a friend or tasting cookies that have been sent as a gift. The notion that this is your only shot at these foods drives you to eat every last bit of the meal or food.

HOW IS DIETING POSSIBLE?

If deprivation backlash is so powerful, how do dieters actually diet at all? Aren't the biological and psychological forces too compelling? Chronic dieters adapt by changing both their mind-set and their responsiveness to inner body cues. This adaptation is known as *restrained eating.* Unfortunately, these changes work against them. In the long run, deprivation backlash still prevails.

Restrained eaters, in essence, are chronic dieters who are preoccupied with dieting and weight control. To stay in control with their food, restrained eaters set up rules that dictate how they should eat, rather than listening to their bodies. Forget *honor your hunger*; instead, they calculate what to eat, choosing foods with their mental brakes on, and second-guessing the needs of their bodies. Their eating appears to be fine until one of their sacred rules is violated. When a rule is broken, so is their restraint—and wham, overeating begins. This has been described as *the what-the-hell effect* by leading researchers in this field Janet Polivy, Ph.D., and C. Peter Herman, Ph.D., from the University of Toronto. And it is *that* phrase, rather than the term restraint eating, that most of our clients relate to! Here's what it means in eating terms:

- The moment a forbidden food is eaten, overeating takes place.
- The moment a calorie level is exceeded, overeating takes place.
- The mere *perception* of breaking a food rule or eating a forbidden food triggers overeating.

Restrained Eating Studies

Studies on restrained eaters have shed a lot of psychological light in the world of dieting. They show how ineffective outlawing particular foods can be, and how it sets you up for overeating. Most restraint studies follow this core procedure:

A short ten-question test called the Restraint Scale is given to identify who the restrained eaters are. (Questions include frequency of dieting, history of weight loss and gain, weekly weight fluctuations, emotional effect of weight fluctuations, effect of "others" on eating, obsessional thinking about food, and guilt feelings about eating.) Then, a "preload" is given—that is, the subjects are "loaded-up" with food *before* the real experiment begins. The preload is a calculated amount of food—and it's usually some sort of set-up to see how the dieters versus nondieters respond in various eating situations. Then the "real" experiment begins.

Here are a couple of particularly significant studies on restrained eaters:

Mind Games—The Counterregulation Effect. One of the classic studies involved fifty-seven female college students at Northwestern University. The students were led to believe that the goal of the study was to evaluate the taste of several ice cream samples. *The actual purpose of the study was to determine how diet thinking might affect eating after drinking milkshakes.* The women were arbitrarily divided into three groups based on the number of eight-ounce milkshakes given (none, one, and two shakes). After drinking the shakes, the subjects were asked to taste and rate three flavors of ice cream. They were allowed to eat as much ice cream as they wanted and "taste-tested" in private to guard against self-consciousness. The researchers saw to it that ample ice cream was provided so that substantial amounts could be eaten without making an appreciable dent in the supply!

Here's what happened. The nondieters naturally regulated their eating; they ate less ice cream in proportion to the amount of milk-shakes consumed. The dieters, however, displayed a dramatic *opposite* behavior. Those who drank two milkshakes ate the *most* ice cream—a "counterregulation" effect. The researchers concluded that forcing the dieters to overeat or "blow their diet" caused them to release their food inhibitions. With inhibition banished, restraint was eliminated and the dieters overate the ice cream.

Perception Affects Eating. A similar study examined the notion of how dieters perceive calories. All subjects were given snacks of chocolate pudding with a substantial calorie difference. One group was given a high-calorie pudding (750 calories) and another was given a lower calorie version (325 calories). But within each of these groups, half of the subjects were told that the pudding was high in calories and half were told that it was low. Then the subjects were given a pseudo taste test. The dieters who *thought* the pudding was high in calories ate more than the dieters who *thought* the pudding was low in calories, by 61 percent! This study illustrates how much power thoughts and perception can have on eating behavior. And once again, when the dieter "blew the diet" (whether actual or perceived), overeating ensued.

The Seesaw Syndrome: Guilt Versus Deprivation

The longer foods are prohibited, the more seductive they become. Consequently, eating these "illegal" foods brings with it a compelling sense of guilt for most dieters. And as the guilt increases, so does food intake. The more deprived you become from dieting and from specific foods, the greater the deprivation backlash. We see this all the time—it's called *the seesaw syndrome*.

When it comes to dieting, feelings of deprivation and guilt work in an opposing manner; like two kids on a seesaw—"what goes up must come down."

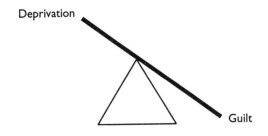

When dieting, as you restrict foods that you enjoy eating, deprivation becomes higher and higher. Meanwhile, in tandem, guilty feelings go down, because you haven't eaten any "bad" foods. But there's a limit to which the seesaw can climb. The level of deprivation rises to its highest point, where you can't bear one more meal, let alone one more day, of restrictive eating. Meanwhile, guilty feelings are at their lowest because you have not eaten any forbidden foods; you've been "good." Since you have no build-up of guilt, you're wide open to allowing some forbidden foods into your life and able to tolerate the beginning feelings of guilt that these foods engender. As you eat the first forbidden food, you begin to feel guilt. That guilt triggers feelings of being "bad," which lead you to more food (the what-the-hell effect), with its accompanying guilt. Now the seesaw looks like a tug-of-war:

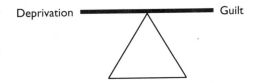

After a while, the guilt continues to build, and in tandem, deprivation begins to recede. As the days go by, you feel worse about breaking your diet rules, and guilt rises to its highest point. Deprivation feelings are virtually nonexistent because you've been eating all the foods that weren't allowed on the diet. Now the seesaw looks like the diagram on the top of the following page.

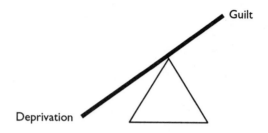

At this point the syndrome repeats itself—up and down, up and down—every time you go from diet to binge, diet to binge. The only way to get off this seesaw is to lighten up and let go of the deprivation. And just as when one kid decides to get off the seesaw, the other is forced to stop playing—when you give yourself permission not to be deprived, you simultaneously let go of the guilt! By giving yourself permission to eat, you stop playing the futile seesaw game.

THE KEY:
UNCONDITIONAL PERMISSION TO EAT

The key to abolishing the pattern of restraint and subsequent over-eating is to give yourself *unconditional* permission to eat. This means:

- Throwing out the preconceived notion that certain foods are "good" and others are "bad." No one food has the power to make you fat or help you become slim.
- Eating what you *really* want. Yes, what you want.
- Eating without obligatory penance. *("Okay, I can have the cheesecake now, but tomorrow I diet.")* These kinds of personal food deals are *not* unconditional.

When you truly free your food choices, without any hidden agenda of restricting them in the future, you eliminate the urgent need to overeat. Yet it's an unsettling prospect to most of our clients, even more frightening than the initial idea of giving up diets.

The Peace Process

Making peace with food means allowing *all* foods into your eating world, so that a choice for chocolate becomes emotionally equal to the choice for a peach. While for years many health professionals have agreed that there should be no forbidden foods, very few will go the distance and say, eat *whatever* you want. Eventually there is a limit imposed. And knowing there is a limit can still impart a food lust of sorts—better eat it now!

Ironically, once you truly know you can eat whatever you want, the intense urge to eat greatly diminishes. The most effective way to instill belief in this fact is to experience eating the very foods you forbid! It becomes self-evident that you can "handle" these foods, or better yet, that they have no magic hold on you or your willpower. Ironically, many of our clients discover that the very foods they prohibited and craved, are no longer desirable once they can be eaten freely. Over and over, we hear stories of how when they were truly allowed to eat certain foods, they discovered, to their surprise, that they really didn't like them to begin with! For example, Molly had relished bakery birthday cakes, but tried not to eat them. She would, however, eventually relent, especially at a party, and power through two or more pieces. But when she decided to make peace with food—and come face-to-face with "official permission"—she found that she did not care for most bakery birthday cakes. She had always eaten them so fast, often on the sly, that she had not truly experienced the taste and texture of the cake! With her newfound permission, Molly took the time to *taste* the cake (whether in the privacy of her home or at a party). She found more often than not that the cakes were stale or bland, and she would not finish a single piece, let alone go for more. Eventually Molly would not settle for cakes that were less than superb. She now often turns down cake at parties—because she wants to, not because she is a diet martyr.

Annie had a similar "taste experience." Her commitment to making peace with food sparked an enthusiasm for taste sensations that had been buried by her restrained eating. Annie gave herself unconditional permission to experience forbidden foods one at a time, day after day, often in preference to all other foods. Annie went through her red licorice phase, her Pop Tart phase, and her mashed potato phase. While in the midst of each phase, she ate the favored food with relish and delight. For some foods, she found that it took a few weeks for the desire to peak and then slowly taper off. For other foods it took longer, and for a few she found that they didn't taste half as good as she had imagined.

To Annie's surprise (and delight), she discovered that once she completed a particular food-freeing phase, *she stopped craving that food, hardly ever thought of it, and sometimes was so sick of it that she never wanted it again!* Removing deprivation from Annie's eating diminished the alluring quality of foods, and instead, put them in a reasonable, rational perspective.

Fears That Hold You Back

Even clients who come ready to give up dieting have a strong resistance against eating whatever they really want. They are terrified. While they feel comfortable learning to *honor their hunger*, they are ready to bolt out the door when we talk about giving unconditional permission to eat what they like.

If people are so afraid to advance to this part of the Intuitive Eating process, why do we insist that it must be explored? Legalizing food is the critical step in changing your relationship with food. It frees you to respond to inner eating signals that have been smothered by negative thoughts and guilt feelings about eating. If you don't truly believe that you can eat whatever food you like, you will continue to feel deprived, ultimately overeat, and be blocked from feeling satisfied with your eating. And when you are not satisfied, you will be on the prowl for more food! When you know the food will be there and allowed, day after day, it doesn't become so important to have it. Food loses its power.

In spite of the knowledge that deprivation leads to backlash eating, many people are apprehensive about making this peace pact with food, in part due to the obstacles described below.

I Won't Stop Eating. At first you may experience an overpowering fear that you won't be able to stop eating a favorite forbidden food.

Just remember that when you know that previously forbidden foods will always be allowed, the urgency to have large quantities of them eventually dissipates. Also research shows that people will tire of eating the same kind of food—it's called habituation. *Habituation studies have shown that the more a person is exposed to a particular food, the less appealing it becomes.* In fact, you may have already witnessed this type of eating in other people. For example, observe the all-you-can-eat buffet dining that is popular in vacation spots such as Las Vegas. On the first day, people typically load up their plates and grab three or four desserts. By the last day, however, they are choosing their food selectively. The novelty has worn off, and they know there is plenty of food.

My entire family (ET) recently encountered the habituation effect when I was working on a two-hundred-recipe cookbook. Whether I was testing salads, appetizers, or casseroles, we eventually tired of eating the same kind of food. This was especially evident while creating the dessert chapter. Not only did we tire of eating sweets, but my husband to this day cannot bear to take a bite of pineapple upside down cake, which was once his favorite! I made that particular cake at least eight times before I decided to give up on that particular recipe.

The only way that *you* will come to believe that you will be able to stop eating is *to go through the food experience, to actually eat.* That's why we are fond of the word "process." This is not about knowledge of food, but rather rebuilding experiences with eating. You cannot have an eating experience through knowledge; rather, you need to go through it, bite by bite. Otherwise it would be like trying to learn how to play the guitar by reading a book on music theory. You may understand the components—but only until you practice and struggle with the strings personally will you truly know how to play. And the more you practice, the more confidence you will have.

Pseudo-Permission: I've Tried It Before. Many of our clients recount that when they "allowed" themselves to eat certain forbidden foods, they still overate and felt out of control. But for most people these foods were never really *unconditionally* allowed; rather, they were only given pseudo-permission. These forbidden foods were actually being eaten with a sense of temporarily breaking the rules, or with a little voice saying "you really shouldn't eat that." The moment that food touched the tongue, feelings of guilt and remorse flooded in. And with these feelings came a conviction to limit these foods in the future and counter this indulgence by "eating right" tomorrow. Although physically eating the food, they were emotionally depriving themselves in the future. And so the cycle was perpetuated. Pseudo-permission does not work—it's only an illusion. Your mouth may be chewing, but your mind is saying, "I shouldn't." Your mind is still on a diet.

A Self-Fulfilling Prophecy. Sometimes just the thought that you will overeat is enough to actually make you do it. Carolyn initially had the strong conviction that white flour would cause her to overeat. She believed that even one bite of a bagel would trigger a binge. And it did. Carolyn had created a self-fulfilling prophecy. She "knew" these foods were fattening; she "knew" she would binge; and she "knew" she would gain weight. Every time she gave in to her craving for white bread, she sincerely told herself that this would be the last time. Of course, she ended up overdoing—the depriving thoughts and feelings, along with her sense of being bad, sent her out of control.

It took a long time before Carolyn was truly able to permit herself to eat foods with white flour, but now she rarely binges on these foods. Every now and then a fleeting, archaic thought of restriction occurs and drags her back to the world of deprivation. And with that thought comes her occasional sense of loss of control. Now, though, she only has a few cookies instead of the whole bag; and this happens once every six months instead of every week. Because Carolyn has had so many positive experiences with foods containing white flour, it has become much easier for her to let go of her restrictive thinking and make peace with these foods.

I Won't Eat Healthfully. In case after case, when people are given free choice and access to all varieties of food after going through the peace process, they end up balancing their intake to include mostly nutritious foods with a smattering of "play foods." As nutritionists, we continue to honor and respect nutrition, but at this point in the Intuitive Eating process, nutrition is not the driving force. If nutrition were the overriding priority now, it would only perpetuate your restrictive thoughts. (It took us years to come to terms with this factor, and it is why nutrition issues are reserved for later in this book.) As you go farther along with the process and all foods are completely allowed, your intuitive signals will give you good advice. But even right now, if you think about eating a hot fudge sundae for every meal, how soon do you think you will be craving something completely opposite, such as a salad or a piece of grilled chicken?

Lack of Self-Trust. A mighty obstacle to making peace with food is a strong lack of self-trust. Most clients say that they trust us and our philosophy. They truly believe that it has worked for "other" clients, but they distrust themselves and are frightened that it won't work for them.

Ironically, the process of giving yourself permission to eat is actually the stepping-stone to rebuilding your trust with food and with yourself. In the beginning, each positive food experience is like a tiny thread. They may be few and far between, and seem insignificant, but eventually the threads form a strand. The strands multiply into strong ropes and finally the ropes become the bridge to a foundation of trust in food and in yourself.

Betsy was gaining weight by the moment when she first came in. She had been on several very restricted diets and was now rebound eating in an out-of-control fashion. After a short time of giving herself permission to eat, she began to find herself eating only *one* candy bar instead of three, which was a major breakthrough. At first these experiences were sporadic and her successes were interspersed with large gaps of bingeing behavior. But Betsy was gradually able to see her successes build upon each other and watch her overeating begin to disappear. Soon she began to redevelop that sense of self-trust that had been eroded by her history of dieting.

For some, the trust issue goes even deeper. Several studies have shown that the regulation of food intake has its foundation in early eating experiences. If as a child your parents took control over most of your eating without respecting your preferences or hunger levels, you easily got the message that you couldn't be trusted with food.

Sarah described this as the push-or-pull-away effect. Her mom was either pushing her to eat, while exerting pressure about Sarah's weight, or pulling food away. At dinnertime, for example, Sarah's mom forced her to clean her plate even when she was full. Sarah remembers coming home from school on several occasions feeling famished and heading for the fridge for a snack. Her mom would chastise her, "You can't be hungry," and forbid her to eat. Consequently, Sarah would sneak food when her mom wasn't looking. By that time, however, hunger was no longer mild, but intense. Sarah would overeat in response to hunger, but she felt guilt from overeating and shame from sneaking the food. And she grew to believe that her mother was right—she couldn't be trusted with food. Wrong!

Don't underestimate the profound impact self-trust can have. Psychoanalyst Erik Erikson, a noted pioneer in human development, explains how critical trust is. According to Erikson, all people must go through a series of stages throughout their lives. The first developmental stage deals with basic trust. During each stage there is a significant issue or crisis that presents itself and must be resolved. If this task is not handled well, a person will continue to struggle with it into adulthood. If food becomes a battleground during this stage, the ability to trust yourself with food becomes tarnished. The you-can't-be-trusted-around-food message becomes compounded if you were put on diets by your parents or your doctor. As an adult, try as you may, you still don't trust yourself. That child can still reside within you, making you fearful of giving yourself permission to eat unconditionally.

Fortunately, Erikson had an optimistic belief that childhood crises can be resolved at any time later in life. If you take back ownership of your eating signals by making peace with food, you can heal one of the most basic trust issues and go on to a healthier relationship with food.

Five Steps to Making Peace with Food

Keep in mind as you read through these steps that it's okay to proceed at a pace with which *you* are comfortable. There is no need to feel overwhelmed by going to the grocery store and buying every single forbidden food—we find that is too big a step and not necessary. It takes time to build up trust in yourself. Before you proceed, please be sure that you are consistently *honoring your hunger*. A ravenous person is bound to overeat regardless of his or her intention.

1. Pay attention to foods that appeal to you and make a list of them.

2. Put a check by the foods you actually do eat, then circle remaining foods that you've been restricting.

3. Give yourself permission to eat one forbidden food from your list, then go to the market and buy this food, or order it at a restaurant.

4. Check in with yourself to see if the food tastes as good as you imagined. If you find that you really like it, continue to give yourself permission to buy or order it.

5. Make sure that you keep enough of the food in your kitchen so that you know it will be there if you want it. Or if that seems too scary, go to a restaurant and order the particular food as often as you like.

Once you've made peace with one food, continue on with your list until all the foods are tried, evaluated, and freed. If your list is quite large, which is possible, we have found that you don't have to experience each and every food listed. Rather, what is important is that you continue this process until you *truly know* you can eat what you want. You will get to a point where you don't have to experience the "proof" by eating.

If these steps seem like too much to handle right now, don't worry. Maybe you can call a ceasefire, that's okay—it's progress. The next chapter will give you some tools to help you loosen up with your food. Just as many peace treaties require a team of negotiators—and time—the next chapter will help you discover powerful allies to help keep the peace with food.

Chapter Eight

PRINCIPLE 4:

Challenge the Food Police

Scream a loud "No" to thoughts in your head that declare you're "good" for eating under 1,000 calories or "bad" because you ate a piece of chocolate cake. The Food Police monitor the unreasonable rules that dieting has created. The police station is housed deep in your psyche and its loudspeaker shouts negative barbs, hopeless phrases, and guilt-provoking indictments. Chasing the Food Police away is a critical step in returning to Intuitive Eating.

I *felt so guilty eating an extra piece of birthday cake that when I felt nauseous for three days, I thought I had earned and deserved this misery. To my surprise, I found out one week later that nausea was not my penance for my eating indulgence—I was pregnant!"*
—A Chronic Dieter

We have become a nation riddled with guilt about how we eat. Even nondieters experience eating angst. In a random survey of 2,075 adults, 45 percent said they feel guilty after eating foods they like! And nearly all of our clients also feel that way—guilty, guilty, guilty.

The thought of stealing or lying would instill a sense of guilt in most people. Yet, most dieters are able to create an equivalent level of guilt when they've eaten french fries or a hot fudge sundae. The quantity of any of these "bad" foods has almost nothing to do with the level of despair that is felt when they are eaten. The first bite often evokes a sense of having failed, or being bad. Eating a "bad" or "illegal" food then becomes a morality issue. The subsequent guilt that builds is enough to initiate a period of overeating that can destroy any previous successful weight loss.

Foods are often described in moralistic terms, independent of dieting: decadent, sinful, tempting—all the words of food fundamentalism and eating morality. Historian Roberta Pollack Seid concluded in her book *Never Too Thin* that our beliefs about food resemble dietary laws of a false religion—we pay homage to dieting and its rules, but it doesn't work.

Since we are a nation that worships the lean body, it easily becomes virtuous to be eating foods associated with slimness and guiltlessness. It is no wonder that dieters have been found to think of food in terms of *absence* of guilt. A major finding in a 1987 study on chronic dieters at the University of Toronto, was that the dieting experience appears to make the guilt-free aspect of foods a key attribute. One in four dieters categorized food using both "guilt" and "no guilt" labels, compared to one out of twenty-five nondieters. Dieters primarily felt guilt for highly caloric, diet-breaking foods.

But dieters don't corner the market in the food guilt department. Nondieters, in the same study, associated guilt with poor nutritional quality of foods. And the media and food companies play a hand in this, tugging at our food consciences, whether or not we are dieting.

Food companies, magazines, and commercials are capitalizing on consumer eating morality with absolving themes, for example:

- Kenny Rogers Roasters' "Eat No Evil" menu
- Guiltless Gourmet (a food company that specializes in fat-free snacks)
- "It's like you dieted and went to heaven" (a magazine ad for Bailey's Light)
- "Butter Paroled, Margarine Charged" (an article in *Eating Well* magazine)

With these daily reminders, it becomes difficult to view eating as simply a normal pleasurable activity; rather, it becomes good or bad, with the societal Food Police chastising each blasphemous bite of food. The Food Police are alive and well—both as a collective cultural voice, and at the individual level, in the thoughts of our clients.

As you embark on your journey to Intuitive Eating, you may encounter your fair share of societal Food Police—from the well-meaning friend, who comments, "How can you eat *that*, I thought you were trying to lose weight," to unsolicited commentary on your eating habits from a stranger. Just because someone makes an inappropriate comment does not make it true! Yet it can shed seeds of doubt as you begin to explore a new eating world that runs counter to the doctrine of fat-phobia orthodoxy in this nation.

Just recently on a vacation, I (ET) experienced an unwelcome Food Police barb. I placed my order at the customized omelet bar, and requested an egg white omelet with mushrooms and *cheese*. The chef nearly gave me hell for my order; he reprimanded, "How can you order an egg white omelet with that fatty cheese, it's loaded with cholesterol." That unsolicited remark would have devastated most of my patients. I was on vacation, and did not feel like defending my consciously placed order. I knew full well what I was doing— I don't miss egg yolks, so why eat them? I'm not crazy about cheese, but since I was pregnant during this vacation, it was one way I was able to get my calcium in since I'm not fond of drinking milk. It was my clients' worst fear personified.

We have found that regardless of the level of inappropriate comments from the collective Food Police—the inner Food Police that reside in the minds of our clients are even harsher. If our nation is being possessed by a food fundamentalism, then certainly no less than a Food Police exorcism will do.

FOOD TALK

In the world of dieting we develop a whole retinue of thoughts that can work against us. Self-awareness, or having the ability to think about our thoughts, distinguishes us from animals. It's also human, however, to let our busy lives lead us from one rote activity to the next without stopping to examine our thoughts. Food thoughts and judgments run rampant through our minds, but how often do we take a moment to focus on them? We're not born with these thoughts. We hear the ideas behind them as we grow up, take them in, and sometimes then adopt them as "well-known" rules which must not be defied.

Here is some of the "knowledge" that prevails in the minds of our clients when they first come to see us:

- Sweets are bad for you.
- I shouldn't eat anything after 6:00 P.M.
- You should take in zero grams of fat.
- Walking three times a week won't do me any good.
- If I eat breakfast, it will just make me eat more throughout the day.
- Dairy products are bad for you.
- I shouldn't have any salt.
- Beans are fattening.
- Bread is fattening.
- Everything is fattening!

Even when these thoughts are evaluated, they stick like glue in the consciousness of the people who think them. Although there has been a great deal of evidence to refute these thoughts, they've become so well entrenched that it often takes years to loosen their hold and replace them with reality. The thoughts themselves can be very damaging and can affect subsequent behavior. These thoughts are called cognitive distortions, and we call the voices that speak these distortions the Food Police.

WHO'S TALKING

There are many ways of looking at personality structure. Psychotherapist and M.D. Eric Berne tells us that the way we feel and act make up what are called *ego states*. If you watch the way a person is standing and listen to his voice, the words he uses, and the views he's stating, you'll be able to detect which ego state he is in. Dr. Berne simply labels these ego states as the Parent, the Adult, and the Child. He believes that at any particular time, you may be in any one of these three ego states and can shift quite easily from one to another. Each ego state can direct the thoughts floating around in your head. You can begin to identify just which one of them is speaking by listening carefully to what is being said.

We have found that in the world of dieting and eating, specific voices crop up from moment to moment which influence how we feel and how we behave. We have extrapolated from Berne's theory of ego structure and identified the following eating voices. There are three that can be primarily destructive: the Food Police, the Nutrition Informant, and the Diet Rebel. But we also can develop powerful allies; these voices are: the Food Anthropologist, the Nurturer, the Rebel Ally, and the Nutrition Ally.

Let's look at each voice—how each can help or harm our thinking process in the world of eating. The following diagrams give an overview of how they interrelate:

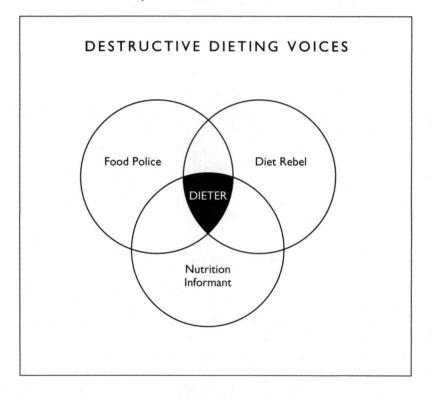

The Food Police

The Food Police is a strong voice that's developed through dieting. It's your inner judge and jury that determines if you are doing "good" or "bad." The Food Police is the sum of all your dieting and food rules, and gets stronger with each diet. It also gets strengthened through new food rules that you may read about in magazines or messages you hear from friends and family. The Food Police is alive and well even when you are not dieting (like a lobbyist positioning his issue during an election year).

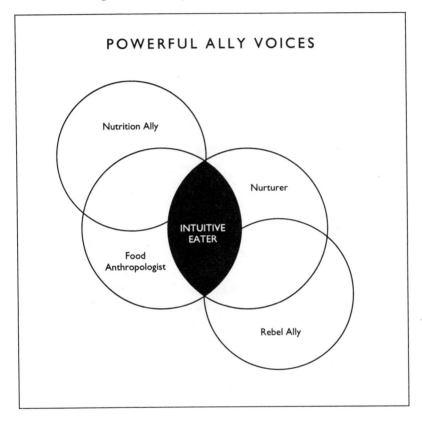

Here are some common rules by which the Food Police may judge your eating actions:

- Don't eat at night (therefore if you eat at night, you are guilty of a violation).
- Better not eat that bagel—it's fattening, too many carbohydrates.
- You didn't exercise today, better not eat dinner.
- It's not time to eat yet—don't have that snack.
- You ate too much (even though it was based on being hungry).

It's important to remember that even when you reject dieting and begin to make peace with food, the Food Police will often surface. But it's not always obvious—just like a weed cut above the surface. A weed that is strongly rooted can easily flourish, even when there are no green tendrils peeking through the soil.

How It Hurts: The Food Police scrutinizes every eating action. It keeps food and your body at war.

How It Helps: *It doesn't!* This is one voice that does not turn into an ally. By identifying its strong presence in your mind, however, you will learn how to challenge its power and loosen its hold on you.

Cyndi had a powerful Food Police voice that criticized her every eating act. She woke up every morning praying for a "good" day, which meant eating only diet foods. But her Food Police voice set impossible standards. Her good day would begin with a light breakfast of grapefruit juice and a small bowl of cereal. On some days her growling stomach would beg for more food—just an extra piece of toast. Cyndi would "cave in" and have a piece of dry rye toast, and her Food Police would shout, "Now you have to skip lunch or dinner." When Cyndi was able to skip lunch, she'd get too hungry and find herself at the vending machine devouring whatever she could afford. Now, once she had officially broken her Food Police rule, she would overeat the rest of the day. In fact, Cyndi's vicious overeating cycle would begin any time she disobeyed her Food Police. It wasn't until Cyndi began to challenge the Food Police voice that her overeating stopped and her weight loss began.

The Nutrition Informant

The Nutrition Informant provides nutrition evidence to keep you in line with dieting. The Nutrition Informant voice may tell you to fastidiously count fat grams, or eat only fat-free foods, often in the name of health. While this may seem innocuous or even healthy, it's a facade.

The Nutrition Informant makes statements like:

- Check those fat grams, anything above one gram of fat is unacceptable.
- Don't eat foods with added sweeteners.

It's not unusual for someone to say, "I've rejected dieting. I truly believe I can eat what I want—and I *want* to start eating healthfully." It's therefore possible to consciously reject dieting, but instead unknowingly continue to diet by embracing nutrition as a politically correct regimen for keeping your weight down.

How It Hurts: This voice colludes with the Food Police. It operates under the guise of health, but it's promoting an unconscious diet. It can be a little difficult to identify because its messages can mimic the sound advice of health authorities.

For example, Kelly declared, "I've made peace with food, I'm never going to diet again, but I'm ready to start eating healthfully." She was actually burned out on exploring "junk foods" which in and of itself was something she never thought she would accomplish!

Here's what happened. One afternoon at work, Kelly got hungry, so she honored her hunger and ate an apple, in the name of "healthy eating." But one hour later, she was hungry again. Her Nutrition Informant voice chimed in with the Food Police telling her, "You shouldn't be hungry—you just had a healthy apple. Wait until you get home to eat." She waited until she arrived at home, and proceeded to devour almost all the food in her pantry out of ravenous hunger. Later, we talked about satisfying snacks including a bagel or bean soup. "But aren't those fattening?" she asked. "The only snacks I thought I should eat were either fresh fruit or cut-up vegetables." Kelly's description sounded like the diet dogma of snacking, yet she did not see it as such, because she was focused on health and had sincerely rejected dieting. Yet one of Kelly's Food Police rules had surfaced: "If you snack, you can't possibly be hungry later." This rule merged with the Nutrition Informant voice, which declared, "If you snack, it should only be raw veggies or fruit because they're good for you and healthy." While Kelly chose the apple in the name of health and nutrition, she had difficulty honoring her true hunger that surfaced only one hour later; because her Food Police and Nutrition Informant voices were overpowering (yet subtle, because she did not recognize them).

How It Can Help: The Nutrition Informant becomes the Nutrition Ally when the Food Police are exiled. The newly emerged Nutrition Ally is interested in healthy eating with *no hidden agenda*. For example, if you were choosing between two brands of cheese that you like equally, the Nutrition Ally would advise choosing the brand with lower fat. It's a choice based on health and pleasure, *not* deprivation or dieting. This voice can help you cut the fat where you won't miss it. We have found that the helpful version of this voice is one of the last to truly appear without being tied into the Food Police. (*Note:* We will address nutrition later in the book. Remember, however, that focusing initially on nutrition can undermine your attempts to be truly free from dieting. It's not that nutrition is not important, but rather that it can be self-defeating in the beginning stages of Intuitive Eating. Remember, we *are* nutritionists and we honor health!)

One distinguishing factor between the Nutrition Ally and the Nutrition Informant is how you *feel* when you respond. If you make, or reject, a food choice in the name of health but feel acquiescent or guilty, then you know the Food Police still have a stronghold on your Nutrition Informant who's guiding your decision.

The Diet Rebel

The voice of the Diet Rebel often bellows loudly in your head. It sounds angry and determined. Here are some typical statements of your internal Diet Rebel:

- You're not going to get me to eat that plain broiled chicken!
- I'll show you, you think I should lose five pounds, huh—I'll put on ten.
- Let's see how many cookies I can stuff in before Mom comes home.
- I can't wait until my husband goes out of town so I can eat whatever I want, without his chastising glares.

How It Hurts: Unfortunately, these rebellious comments reside in your head, because you're usually too scared to confront your "space invaders" and tell them to bug off. Feeling powerless over their messages, you feel resigned to merely possessing the thoughts you wish you could say out loud, and then end up carrying out their "threats" just to spite them.

Janie had a strong Diet Rebel voice. Every time her mother put her on a diet as a child, Janie's sneak-eating would escalate. The Diet Rebel voice was Janie's primary guiding force as a child and as an adult. Janie would hang out at her friends' homes so she could eat as much of their treats as she could stuff in her mouth. Overweight as a child, Janie became morbidly obese as an adult. When her ex-husband carried on the parental diet messages, Janie's silent Diet Rebel became loud and angry. It was her "forget-you" inner voice that directed her to go against any rules imposed upon her, which resulted in overeating. Janie's boundaries were being invaded everywhere she turned. In order to protect her autonomy, Janie's Diet Rebel was overpowering all other voices to help keep her independent. Yet it only ended up in private food riots of overeating.

Unfortunately, when the Diet Rebel rules the roost, self-destruction always ensues. Rebellious behavior often has no limits, and severe overeating is usually the result. How often does the Diet Rebel break forth in your thoughts? How often do you feel compelled to follow its directions, because you're so angry at the Food Police in your life imposing their dieting rules on you?

How It Can Help: You can turn your Diet Rebel into the Rebel Ally. Use the Rebel Ally to help you protect your boundaries against anyone who invades your eating space. *Use your mouth for words instead of food* in a direct but polite manner—it's surprising how powerful it can make you feel, while giving you a tremendous release.

- Ask your family members to stay out of your food choices or amounts. For example: "Aunt Carolyn, please don't push that second portion on me. I'm full, thank you." Or, "No thanks, Mom, I don't like macaroni and cheese. You know I've never liked macaroni and cheese."
- Tell your family and your friends and people on the street that they may not make comments about your body. For example: "Dad—my body is *my* business!" Or, "Joey, you have no right to comment about my weight."

The Food Anthropologist

The Food Anthropologist is simply the neutral observer. This is the voice that makes observations *without* making judgment. It's a neutral voice that takes note of your thoughts and actions with respect to your food world, without an indictment—just like an anthropologist would observe an individual or culture. It's the voice that will let you explore and discover. The Food Anthropologist will help pave the way to the world of Intuitive Eating. For example, noticing when you're hungry or full, what you eat, the time of day, and what you're thinking, are some of the actions of the Food Anthropologist. This voice simply observes and shows you how to interact with food both behaviorally and inwardly. The advantage to developing this voice is that only *you* know what you feel and think.

The statements of the Food Anthropologist are purely observational such as:

- I skipped breakfast and was ravenous at 2:00 P.M.
- I ate ten cookies. (No judgment here, just the facts.)
- I experienced guilt after eating dessert with dinner. (No condescending statements, just an observation of how you felt.)

One easy way to call your inner Food Anthropologist into action is to keep a food journal. Sometimes simply noting the time of day and what you ate can give you some interesting clues about what drives your eating. Or note your thoughts before and after you eat. Do they affect how you *feel*? Does how you feel affect how you behave or eat? If so, how? Consider this one big experiment, *not a tool for judgment*.

Many of our clients have had negative experiences with food journals because it was a requirement of past diets. But in those cases the food journal was used as evidence to convict bad eating! We use the food journal only as a learning tool. Yet in spite of the fact that we stress this, our first-time clients still expect to get verbally beaten-up upon their return visit for any "eating indiscretion" or violation. Remember, this is not a tool of the Food Police, but a tool to help you access the Food Anthropologist.

How It Helps: The Food Anthropologist can help you sort through the facts rather than letting you get caught up in the emotionally labile experience of eating. It keeps you in touch with your inner signals—biologically and psychologically. We often play the role of the Food Anthropologist with our clients until they can build their own voice. (It can be hard to be just neutral when you've had a critical voice harping on every food choice.) The Food Anthropologist can help find the loopholes in your thinking, similar to the way a sharp attorney can find the loopholes in a contract. But using this voice does take practice.

The Nurturer

The Nurturer's voice is soft and gentle and has the soothing quality that might be associated with the voice of a loving grandparent or best friend. It has the ability to reassure you that you're okay and that everything will turn out fine. It never scolds or pressures. It's not critical or judgmental. Instead, it is (or can be) the vehicle for most of the positive self-talk in your head.

Here are some of the messages you might hear from the Nurturer in your head:

- It's okay to have a cookie. Eating a cookie is normal.
- I really overate today. I wonder what I was feeling that could have made me need more food to comfort myself?
- When I take care of myself, I feel great.
- I'm doing so well this week. There were only a few times I didn't honor my hunger signals.
- I'm getting more in touch with myself every day.
- Losing weight is a long, slow process, and I'm having many successes along the way.

Alice is a mother who usually knows just the right thing to say to her children to make them feel safe and secure. But for many years, Alice had not learned to speak to herself kindly about her weight problem. The voice of the Food Police punished her severely through all of her diets. On her journey to becoming an Intuitive Eater, Alice learned to counter the messages of the Food Police with the supportive messages of the Nurturer. She listened to herself speak to her family and realized that the voice she used when speaking to them was the same voice she needed to comfort herself.

Alice learned to be understanding of the stumbling blocks in her path and to patiently reassure herself that she was in the midst of a process. When she would have difficulty honoring her hunger, she'd gently ask herself what was bothering her and what she really needed instead of food. When she found herself craving a food she had restricted on one of her many diets, the Nurturer gave her permission to eat that food.

How It Helps: When you get in touch with the Nurturer inside your head, you will experience one of the most significant tools to becoming an Intuitive Eater. The Nurturer will be there for you to help you to challenge the Food Police and support you through this process. The Nurturer provides coping statements for the harsh zingers that the Food Police and the Diet Rebel can throw.

The Intuitive Eater

The Intuitive Eater speaks your gut reactions. You were born as an Intuitive Eater, but this persona has probably been suppressed for most of your life by the voices of the Food Police (prevailing in your family and in society), the Diet Rebel, and the Nutrition Informant.

The Intuitive Eater is a compilation of the positive voices of the Food Anthropologist, who is able to observe your eating behavior neutrally, and the Nurturer, who holds you with supportive statements to get you through the tough times, as well as the Rebel Ally and the Nutrition Ally. The Intuitive Eater knows how to argue the negative voices out of your head. For example, it knows how to challenge the distorted messages of the Food Police and how to get the Rebel Ally to speak out loud to fend off the boundary invaders.

The Intuitive Eater might say some of the following things:

- That little rumble in my stomach means I'm hungry and need to eat.
- What do I feel like eating for dinner tonight? What sounds good to me?
- It feels so good to be out of that dieting prison.

These statements all tell you about your gut reactions. They're instinctual and hit you out of nowhere, without your having to think about them. You'll find that you'll be in the midst of a meal and the Intuitive Eater knows that you're satisfied. Or you'll be doing some writing and a hunger pang will emerge. Or maybe your eyes lock onto the food on the menu that connects with your craving. When you have reached the last stages of your path to Intuitive Eating, the Intuitive Eater, rather than the Dieter, will prevail most of the time. But there will be times when you find that you'll need to evoke one or all of the positive eating voices to help you get centered and in touch with your Intuitive Eater once again. There are no rigid rules in this process. Diets are rigid—Intuitive Eating is fluid and adapts to the many changes in your life. Go with the flow without trying to control it.

The integrated Intuitive Eater honors gut reactions, whether they are biological, pleasure-based, or self-protective. The *Intuitive Eater is a team player* and can draw from the voices of the Nurturer, the Food Anthropologist, and the positive traits of both the Diet Rebel and the Nutrition Informant.

EATING VOICES: HOW THEY EMERGE AND EVOLVE

Each of the eating voices may prevail at different times. Some of the voices were there at birth but many have become buried. Others were instilled by family and society. And some need to be learned and developed to become an Intuitive Eater.

You're born with the innate ability to sense when you're hungry and full. These are primitive signals and are the basis for the emerging Intuitive Eater, which is operating in the toddler as he or she starts eating solid food. The Intuitive Eater tells you what you like and what you don't like. If your parents are not sensitive to your signals, you may learn to mistrust these signals and ultimately lose touch with them.

If you happen to live in a family that has weight and eating issues, you may have your first experience with the voice of the Food Police when you are still very young. You may be told to stop eating so much or be restricted from eating certain foods. It doesn't take long before you internalize those negative messages, and create your own powerful Food Police. If, on the other hand, you're lucky enough to have a family who is not invasive, making no food or body judgments, you may not encounter the Food Police until you start school, or even until you become a teen reading magazines and listening to your friends talk. If the pressure to be thin is strong

	SUMMARY: HOW THE FOOD VOICES HELP OR HARM	
Voice	How It Harms	How It Helps
Food Police	Causes guilt and food worry. Full of judgment. Keeps you in the dieting world, and out of touch with inner cues of eating.	It doesn't.
Nutrition Informant	Uses nutrition as a vehicle to keep you dieting.	Once uncoupled from the Food Police, it becomes the *Nutrition Ally* and can help you make healthy food choices without guilt.
Diet Rebel	Usually results in overeating, self-sabotage.	When the Diet Rebel becomes the *Rebel Ally*, it can help you guard your food turf/ boundaries.
Food Anthropologist	It doesn't.	A neutral observer that can give you a distant perspective into your eating world. Nonjudgmental. Keeps you in touch with your inner signals— biologically and psychologically.
Nurturer	It doesn't.	Helps to disarm the verbal assault from the Food Police. Gets you through the tough times.

in your community, you are at risk of making the Food Police messages your own at any time in your life. And the Nutrition Informant constantly feeds nutrition information about food to the Food Police.

The voice of the Diet Rebel will crop up soon after you've encountered the Food Police. They usually go hand in hand. The Food Police come in and invade your boundaries by interfering with your intuitive biological and food preference signals. In order to protect your private space, the Diet Rebel feeds you "forget-you" messages that not only counter the Food Police but often send you off into a one-person food riot.

The Food Anthropologist will help give you a neutral perspective. For some individuals, interaction with this voice is often the first nonjudgmental, nonnegative encounter with food.

The Nurturer can get you through outside abuse and your own self-defeating behavior if you have access to its positive voice. If your family has given you a sense that you are competent and adequate and has modeled positive ways of coping, you may easily find the voice of your nurturer to combat the societal voices of the Food Police. If, however, your family has colluded with society and you have grown up with criticism and judgment, the Nurturer will have to be found elsewhere. Sometimes a grandparent, aunt or uncle, or dear friend may teach you how to speak kindly to yourself. For some, seeking help from a psychotherapist or dietitian may be the first experience with learning positive self-talk. However you learn to bring forth the voice of the Nurturer, this is a critical step in becoming an Intuitive Eater. You must make it available to yourself so you can buffer the negative voices which bombard you without notice and impede your progress.

And finally, you find yourself back at that place where the Intuitive Eater is running the show. The Intuitive Eater integrates the voices of the Nurturer, the Food Anthropologist, the Nutrition Ally, and the Rebel Ally. The Intuitive Eater knows when your biological signals are calling; it tells you what you need and want, and with guidance from the other positive voices helps you make adult, neutral decisions about how you will take care of yourself.

Let's now take an eating situation and listen for the dialogue of voices that can affect its outcome.

You've been invited to dinner at the home of a gourmet cook. Many appetizers will be served during the cocktail hour, and later

*a spectacular dinner will be placed before you. Unfortunately, you
arrive at the party in an overhungry state.*

THE FOOD POLICE: You'd better be careful of what you eat. Everything
is fattening. Don't touch the appetizers. If you even taste that
little quiche you're a goner. And you can be sure you'll be
tempted with lots of rich desserts. Watch out!

THE NUTRITION INFORMANT: You shouldn't have any cheese because
there's too much fat in it, and the salt will make you feel bloated.
You can only eat the raw veggies.

THE DIET REBEL: Nobody is going to tell me what I can eat at this party.
I hate that stupid diet. I've had to succumb to cardboard crackers
and diet cottage cheese. Well not tonight. I'm going to get my
fill of these amazing foods. I don't care what happens to my
diet. I don't care if I'm fat. I'll show my wife what she can do
with comments about my weight.

THE FOOD ANTHROPOLOGIST: Look at the interesting array of appetizers.
A lot of them look great. You're overly hungry—better eat something, or you'll probably overeat at dinner.

THE NUTRITION ALLY: I don't think I'll have any cheese or fried appetizers
tonight. I'd rather have some crab and veggies now and save
the fat for the main meal.

THE NURTURER: This food looks terrific. I want to taste *everything*.
It's scary to feel such an overwhelming desire to devour these
appetizers. That's okay; it's normal to feel this way when you're
ravenous. This isn't the usual situation, and I'm human.

THE INTUITIVE EATER: I'm starving. But I think I'll pace myself, so I
won't feel too full to enjoy the dinner later. Let's see, of all the
appetizers, which look the best? Oh, I haven't had rumaki in a
long time—that looks good, and so does the baked brie. I think
I'll try them both. The brie is great, but the bacon is undercooked
on the rumaki—think I'll just leave it and taste the stuffed mushrooms.

    (*Halfway through dinner.*) This is delicious, but I'm starting
to feel full. One more bite, and I'll feel satisfied. I feel great
getting to eat anything I like and leaving half of it (without feeling
deprived).

THE REBEL ALLY: (*to the hostess*) The dinner is delicious, but I'm quite
full and couldn't eat another helping. Thanks, anyway.

SELF-TALK: SPECIAL ARSENAL
FOR CHALLENGING FOOD POLICE

Identifying the inner eating voices is useful for challenging the Food Police. But this powerfully negative voice requires more ammunition. The Food Police can throw many tricks that require special attention—especially in the thought process department.

When working with dieters in our offices, we have seen over and over that there is actually a middle step between the initial dieting thought and subsequent eating behavior. We have found that the inner dieting myths (which are cognitive distortions) lead to feeling bad when the self-imposed dieting rules are broken. This concept is widely accepted and well explained by Dr. Albert Ellis and Dr. Robert A. Harper, highly respected pioneers in the field of rational-emotive psychotherapy, a system of psychotherapy which deals with the effect of our thoughts on our feelings and then our behaviors.

According to Ellis and Harper, we routinely flood our heads with crazy notions as well as sane and rational messages. These thought processes are called internalized sentences or *self-talk*. Negative self-talk often makes us feel despair. The feeling of despair can trigger sabotaging behaviors. They believe that if we challenge the "nonsense" in our heads, we'll end up feeling better. When we feel better, we'll act better. In a review of hundreds of research studies of this type of therapy, it has been shown that if we can first change our *beliefs*, our feelings and behaviors will also change in a chainlike reaction. Therefore, it makes sense to examine our food or diet beliefs and the influence they can have.

Here's a favorite story that illustrates this principle. Let's say that you are a dieter who has been carefully following your diet for several weeks. Your diet is low-fat and prohibits any kind of sugary, fatty desserts. You decide that you're going to visit your grandmother, whom you haven't seen for a while. You walk into Grandma's house and the first thing that strikes you is the enticing aroma of chocolate brownies hot out of the oven.

Here are the *food beliefs* and *thoughts* that might fill your head:

- I've been so good on my diet the last few weeks.
- I haven't had any ice cream or candy or cookies.

- I'd sure love to have one of those brownies, but I can't—I shouldn't—I won't!
- If I have a brownie, I'll blow my diet.
- I won't be able to stop eating the brownies.
- Oh, maybe just one will be okay.

You eat the brownie.

- Oh, no—I shouldn't have done that.
- That was really stupid.
- I have no willpower.
- I'm going to be out of control.
- It's all my fault that I'm fat.
- Will I ever be able to lose weight?

Now, let's sense what you are *feeling:*

- Disappointment
- Fear of future deprivation
- Sadness
- Fear of being out of control
- Despair

Typical eating *behavior* that follows will be something like this:

- You slowly take a second brownie,
- . . . and a third brownie.
- Before you know it, you've gobbled up the whole plateful.
- You collapse on the couch, stuffed and miserable, and fall right to sleep.

Now, let's see how challenging and then changing your basic food beliefs can change your feelings and your behavior. The *beliefs* and *thoughts:*

- I'm so glad I gave up dieting.
- I can eat anything I want, any time I want.
- I'd sure love to have one of those brownies.

You eat the brownie.

- Boy, was that delicious.
- I'm satisfied with just this one.

- There's nothing like Grandma's home-baked chocolate brownies.

And now the *feelings:*

- Satisfaction
- Pleasure
- Contentment (no worry about future deprivation)

And the *behavior:*

- You leave the rest of the brownies on the plate.
- You put the plate of brownies on the kitchen counter.
- You're free to enjoy the afternoon with Grandma without another thought about the brownie.

Andrea is a college student who had been suffering from years of low self-esteem associated with her dieting failures. For a short time, she actually became bulimic when she saw no other way to control the bingeing that inevitably followed her dieting "falls from grace." Andrea was an expert at telling herself that carbohydrates were bad and that even a few grams of fat in a day would mar her "good" eating behavior (*belief*). As soon as these *thoughts* formed in her head, she *felt* bad the moment she would eat carbohydrates. The conflict between her restrictive thoughts and her craving for the forbidden food always created angry and hateful feelings. When she *felt* bad in her mode of shaky "willpower," she was off and running to her latest eating disaster (*behavior*).

As soon as Andrea succumbed to her natural desires to eat that food, the system of negative thinking led to negative feelings which led to negative behavior.

Andrea has learned to check her food thoughts as soon as they arise. Old diet rules and thoughts get challenged immediately. Because she is free from distorted dieting thoughts, she feels better about herself and eating. Instead of feeling bad about wanting french fries or ice cream, she feels great about her new relationship with food. And you guessed it—her bingeing days are over.

NEGATIVE SELF-TALK
(AND HOW TO CHANGE IT)

*"... for there is nothing either good or bad but thinking
makes it so. To me it is a prison ..."*

—*Hamlet*

When diet thoughts are irrational or distorted, negative feelings
escalate exponentially. As a result, eating behavior can end up being
extreme and destructive. It's the classic case of perception becoming
reality. Therefore, to change our "food reality," we need to replace
the irrational thinking with rational thoughts. This in turn helps to
moderate our feelings and then our behavior.

To get rid of distorted diet thoughts, you first need to identify
irrational thinking. Ask yourself:

- Am I having *repetitive* and *intense* feelings? (This is a clue
that you need to challenge your thoughts.)
- What am I *thinking* that's leading me to feel this way?
(What are you saying to yourself?)
- What is true or correct about this belief? What is false?
(Examine and confront the *distorted* beliefs that support this
thinking. Your Food Anthropologist voice can be very helpful
here.)

Once you have uncovered your distorted beliefs, you need to
replace them with thoughts and beliefs that are more rational and
reasonable. Here's one example, but the remainder of this chapter
will show you how to do this in various ways.

Replace this distorted thought:	With a more rational thought:
Every time I eat pizza, I'm much fatter the next day.	I am salt-sensitive. Since pizza is pretty salty, I'm most likely bloated. This isn't fat—it's just water retention. It's temporary.

Irrational beliefs often present themselves to us through negative
self-talk. Let's examine the various types of negative thinking and

how you can recognize their signs before they drag you into the ditches of overeating.

Dichotomous Thinking

When I furnished my first office (ER), I purposely chose gray fabric for the couches. I decided that it was a symbolic gesture to help my patients get away from the "black-and-white" thinking that usually coexists with the diet mentality. Here are some typical examples of dichotomous thinking: When you get on the scale in the morning and it drops a pound, you say that you've been "good." If it goes up a pound, you're "bad." When you're dieting, you think in terms of "all or nothing." You're not allowed to have any cookies, and if you eat one, you think and feel that you must finish them all. With dichotomous thinking come black-and-white behaviors. Here are some typical eating examples:

- Eating none or eating all
- Never eating snacks or always eating snacks
- Always eating alone or partying all of the time

Dichotomous or black-and-white thinking can be dangerous and is often based on the premise of achieving perfection. It gives you only two alternatives, one of which is usually neither attainable nor maintainable. The other then tends to be the black hole in which you inevitably fall after failing to get to the first. You set your sights too high, constantly chasing an ideal that you can grasp only moments at a time. When the standard for being okay is this lofty, you're destined to feel lousy most of the time. And we know that when you feel lousy, you're bound to end up going off the deep end in your eating behavior.

For example, Hillary is a client who set herself up for failure by thinking in a black-and-white manner. She would give herself permission to eat only when she felt ravenous. If she ate when just moderately hungry, she would consider it overeating. As a result of thinking that she had "blown it" when she didn't meet her "starving standard," she would feel awful and then go into a binge.

When you think in terms of how good or bad your eating is or how fat or thin your body is, you can end up judging your self-worth based on these thoughts. If you begin to feel that you're a bad person, you're likely to create self-punishing behaviors.

Rae is a young woman who set up perfectionistic standards in her eating style throughout her high school days. She never allowed herself to eat anything with sugar, artificial sweeteners, salt, or fat in it. As a result, she consistently maintained a super thin, even unhealthy, weight. When Rae got to college and was away from the familiarity of home, she found that her standards were becoming impossible to keep up. As soon as she began to expand her food choices as a result of availability, temptation, and peer pressure, things began to fall apart for Rae. As a dichotomous thinker, her thoughts began to run like this:

- The only correct way to eat is the way I ate in high school.
- This new kind of eating is bad and will make me fat.
- I've lost my willpower to eat in the right way.
- The only way I can eat now is wrong.
- That's bad, I'm bad, and I deserve to feel bad.

Rae ultimately began to binge as a result of her dichotomous thinking and was willing to acknowledge that much of her bingeing behavior was done as a way to punish herself for her "bad" acts. The bingeing made her feel increasingly worse, but, ironically, this was okay with her as she felt that she deserved the punishment. Rae ended up gaining sixty pounds and is only now learning to change her thinking. She's stopped talking to herself negatively, is beginning to feel better, has stopped punishing herself with bingeing, and is slowly losing the excess weight.

How do you get out of the dichotomous-thinking trap?

Go for the Gray. Gray may seem to be a dull color, while black and white are dramatic extremes. In the world of eating, however, going for the gray can give you a rainbow of choices. Give up the notion that you must eat in an all-or-nothing fashion. Let go of your old black-and-white dieting rules. Allow yourself to eat the foods that were *always* restricted, while checking your thoughts to be sure that they support your choices.

You'll find that the thrill of being in the white area of diet restriction is gone, but so is the misery of being in the black area of out-of-control behavior.

Absolutist Thinking

When you think in this way, you believe that one behavior will absolutely, irrevocably result in a second behavior. This is considered magical thinking, because in reality, you can't and don't control life in this way. It leads you to believe that you "must" act in a certain way or else something "awful" will happen.

In the world of eating, absolutist thinking will lead you to statements like the following: "I *must* eat perfectly these next two months or else I won't lose enough weight for my daughter's wedding, and that would be *awful*." You don't really have any proof that eating "perfectly" will actually cause you to lose "enough" weight. You're not even sure what "enough" weight actually means. And you really can't define this "awful" state that you imagine. You end up feeling frantic trying to eat perfectly, and then, of course, eat imperfectly. Fearing that you won't lose enough weight makes you more anxious and believing that will be awful turns you into a wreck. The result, of course, of all these absolute thoughts and anxious feelings, is destructive overeating behavior, which leads you to the opposite end of what you wished. You might even *gain* weight before the wedding and feel all the worse.

How do you get away from absolutist thinking?

Banish the Absolutes and Replace Them with Permissive Statements. Carefully listen for the "absolute" words that you use. Get rid of the *musts, oughts, shoulds, need to's, supposed to's,* and *have to's.* Every time you think that you *must* go on a diet, or you *need* to lose ten pounds before the reunion, or you *ought* to have a light lunch like a salad and tea, or you *shouldn't* eat before you go to bed, stop yourself and replace those thoughts. Those kinds of words and thoughts will only cause you anxiety about not being able to carry out the command. Thinking in this absolute way has no guarantee of resulting in the behavior you desire and is likely to create self-sabotaging behavior. In fact, it's fairly sure to make the result *awful*, which is just what you're trying to avoid.

Use words such as *can, is okay,* and *may.* Give yourself permissive statements such as:

- It's okay if I don't lose weight before the wedding.
- I can eat whenever I'm hungry.
- If I want, I can eat whatever foods I like.
- I can have anything that looks good to me.

Catastrophic Thinking

Each time that you think in exaggerated ways, you create miserable feelings for yourself, and, once again, compensate by extreme behaviors. The following are examples of catastrophic thoughts:

- I'll never be thin.
- It's hopeless.
- I'll never get a boyfriend or a job at this weight.
- My life is ruined, because I'm so fat.
- If I let myself eat candy bars and fries, I'll eat them forever.

This kind of thinking is a real set-up. It makes a bad situation worse and ties all of your future successes in life to your ability to eat in a particular way or to losing weight. You tell yourself that all your happiness hinges on your eating and your body. If that is your premise, then you're bound to feel even more unhappy than you are at the moment. You may be desperately unhappy about your weight right now, but you may become despairing by catastrophizing your bleak future.

Marion is a highly successful screenwriter who owns her own home and has many devoted friends and two loving dogs. But Marion feeds herself a daily litany of catastrophic thoughts. Because she's overweight, she tells herself that she'll never get married, never have children, and never be happy. Looking forward to this negative self-created future only makes her feel miserable and causes her to overeat to comfort herself.

How do you get away from catastrophic thinking?

Climb Out of the Abyss. Replace your exaggerated thoughts with thinking which is more positive and accurate. Treat yourself to hopeful, coping statements. Marion is learning to nurture herself by telling herself that many overweight people find spouses who love them as they are. She's practicing positive self-talk that confirms her current as well as her future happiness. As a result, Marion is eating less and is accepting her weight. She's actually lost weight and knows that she'll never return to her former highest weight, which she had reached at the height of her negative self-talk.

Pessimistic Thinking, or "The Cup Is Half Empty"

People who view the world in this way tend to see every situation in its worst-case scenario. They usually think that life is terrible, that they don't have enough of what they want, and that everything that they do is wrong. They're highly critical and blameful, not only of themselves but of others.

Bonnie walks into the office each week with a scowl. She complains about her husband and her job and says that her children are driving her crazy. She begins each session with accounts of how terrible her week has been and how badly she has "blown" her eating. Bonnie would evaluate the cup as half empty. This kind of negative thinking is insidious and often goes unnoticed by the participant. It needs to be pointed out on a regular basis, so the person can reevaluate her thought processes and see that it only leads to a pervasive sense of unhappiness. It also perpetuates self-destructive behaviors. A person who thinks this way has great difficulty appreciating her small successes. She often even misses them and tends to condemn her progress.

How do you get away from pessimistic thinking?

Half-Empty	Half-Full
1. I had a terrible week.	1. I had some success this week.
2. I overate so many times.	2. I had many times when I honored my hunger.
3. All I ate was sweets.	3. I had more sweets than I wished, but I had lots of other foods, too.
4. I feel so fat.	4. I'm feeling better about myself.
5. I'm such a failure.	5. I'm doing better little by little.

Make the Cup Half Full. The most obvious way to heal cup-is-half-empty thinking is to consciously catch each of your negative statements and replace the words with more positive ones.

After you have done this consciously for a while, you'll find that you hear your own negative thoughts transform into more positive words. You will also become sensitive to how hard you've been on yourself. Once you begin to see the world in terms of the cup being half full, you'll find that your daily dose of happy moments increases regularly. Soon you'll see many of your negative eating habits disappear along with the negative thoughts.

Linear Thinking

If you've been on even one diet, you'll know that diet thinking goes in one straight line. You begin at your initial weight, and all you can think about is getting to your goal weight. You follow a very specific plan that allows for no deviations. It's like trying to walk along the white line in the middle of the highway to get to your destination. If you put one foot in front of the other in perfect style, you'll successfully make it to the end. If you accidentally step off the line for even a moment, you're likely to be a highway disaster. We tend to be a society of linear thinkers. We want to get to the goal without appreciating the means. We're success-oriented and rarely stop long enough to check out the scenery along the way.

Here are some examples of linear thinking that can set you up:

- All that is important is that I lose this weight.
- The faster I lose weight, the more successful I am.
- To be successful I must reach my goal weight by the specified target date.
- I will lose two pounds per week with no fluctuations.

How do you get away from linear thinking?

Switch to Process Thinking. The cure for linear thinking is *process thinking*, which focuses on continual change and learning rather than just the end result. If you start thinking in terms of what you can learn along the way, and accept that there will be many ups and downs, you will go forward. By becoming a process-thinker, you will enjoy the opportunity to enrich many aspects of your life while you're recreating your relationship with food. Process thinking will help you become more sensitive to your intuitive eating signals, rather than the endpoints such as how much you ate today.

Here are some examples of process thinking:

- This was a rough week. But I learned some new things about myself that will help me make changes in the future.
- My weight loss seems to come in spurts. Now and then I even gain a little, but it's all part of the process. Our bodies do not behave like machines with linear results.
- I ate more than I wanted to at the restaurant tonight, especially the dessert. But I learned that giving myself permission to eat dessert took away the urgency to have sweets again. Usually I would have binged when I got home, alone.

SELF-AWARENESS: THE ULTIMATE WEAPON AGAINST THE FOOD POLICE

The next time you see yourself eating in a way that feels uncomfortable, unsatisfying, or even out of control, give yourself the gift of remembering what you were thinking just before you took the first bite of food. Examine that thought and challenge it. As you get more adept at the Intuitive Eating process, you'll be able to catch these food thoughts before they make you feel bad or cause undesirable behavior.

Become self-aware. Pay attention to the food talk that inevitably arises when you approach any eating situation. Listen for the different voices that can either serve as your support or saboteur.

Banish the Food Police that keep you from making your peace with food. Challenge the pseudo-nutrition thoughts that come from the Nutrition Informant. Observe your eating through the eyes and voice of your Food Anthropologist and allow it to guide you sensibly. Speak out loud the thoughts of your Rebel Ally so you don't use food to take care of you. The real protection will come from your

Nurturer, who knows just how to soothe you and get through tough situations. And finally, become acutely sensitive to the positive voices that comprise your Intuitive Eater. It was there when you were born. Discard the layers of negative voices that have buried it so deeply that it seemed lost forever. By listening to your instinctual signals, you'll have the opportunity to form a healthy relationship with food.

Chapter Nine

PRINCIPLE 5:

Feel Your Fullness

Listen for the body signals that tell you you are no longer hungry. Observe the signs that show you're comfortably full. Pause in the middle of eating and ask yourself how the food tastes, and what your current fullness level is.

The vast majority of chronic dieters we have worked with belong to the clean-plate club. And most of them say that they've tried not to eat everything. It may seem that an obvious step to weight loss is to respect your fullness, rather than to habitually clean your plate. Yet leaving food can be difficult to achieve, especially for the chronic dieter.

Dieting instills a license to eat only at mealtime—when it is "legal." Ironically, this sense of entitlement reinforces a clean-your-plate mentality. This is particularly true for our clients who have sipped on over-the-counter liquid diets, such as Slim-Fast. (Liquid diet programs typically have you drink a "beverage-meal" for breakfast and lunch, and then "allow you to eat a sensible dinner" of "real" food.) Naturally, most of our patients practically licked their plates clean when given the opportunity to eat their one real meal. It's not that they overate; rather they ate *all* of their precise and "entitled" portions.

Other diet plans using regular food typically offer small portions at meals. This, too, encourages you to eat while you can. Who would leave any morsel of food when quantities are meager? For example, even frozen diet meals hover at about 300 calories (and often less), which usually leaves you less than satisfied. In fact, there is a new trend of frozen diet entrees offering even fewer calories—closer to

200 calories per package. This type of eating hardly fosters getting in touch with your inner eating signals, especially signals of satiety. Instead, you eat it all.

Perhaps you've tossed your diet plans out years ago, but now carefully count fat grams. You may find, however, that you clean your plate when it comes to eating fat-free foods. We've had several clients eat an entire package of fat-free chocolate cake (or other fat-free goodies) with carefree abandonment because of the entitlement factor. They would rationalize that "There's no fat so I can eat as much as I want." Unfortunately, fat-free is not necessarily calorie-free. But the calories wouldn't even be an issue if people were respecting their fullness level.

Of course, other factors can easily condition you to polish off every crumb on your plate, including:

- Having been taught to finish everything on your plate by well-meaning parents.
- Respecting economics and the value of food—thou shall not waste. Remember, however, that either way the food can be wasted; in the case of chronically eating more than you need, it becomes an issue of w-a-i-s-t.
- Having an ingrained habit of eating to completion. Out of sheer habit you finish an entire plate of food, or a *whole* hamburger, or a *whole* bag of chips, regardless of how hungry or full you are. This is a reliance on external cues. You stop eating when the food is *gone*, regardless of the size of the initial portion.
- Beginning a meal (or snack) in an overly ravenous state. In this state, eating intensity is revved-up and it's all too easy to bypass normal satiety cues.

Even if you don't clean your plate, it's still possible that you may be overeating, or bypassing your comfortable satiety level. With our clients who don't clean their plates, we have often discovered that while there may still be food left on the plate, it took an *uncomfortable* level of fullness to get them to stop eating. The problem is the inability to recognize comfortable satiety or to respect fullness.

THE KEY TO RESPECTING FULLNESS

Respecting fullness, or the ability to stop eating because you have had enough to eat biologically, hinges critically on giving yourself unconditional permission to eat (Principle Three: Make Peace with Food). How can you or any dieter expect to leave food on your plate if you believe that you won't be able to eat that particular food or meal again? Unless you truly give yourself permission to eat again when you are hungry, or to have access to that particular food, respecting fullness simply becomes a dogmatic dieting exercise without roots. It won't take hold. The Intuitive Eater in training learns to stop eating when he or she has had just enough to fill the stomach comfortably without being overfull. It's easier to stop eating at this point and leave food behind, when you *know* you can eat it again later.

RECOGNIZING COMFORTABLE SATIETY

We are surprised at how often our clients do not know what comfortable satiety feels like. Oh yes, they can usually describe with great detail how overeating or being overstuffed feels. But knowledge of what comfortable satiety feels like is often illusive, especially to the chronic dieter. Yet, if you do not know what comfortable satiety feels like, how can you expect to achieve it? It's like trying to shoot at a target without ever seeing it, or knowing where it resides. When respecting fullness is the target, it could easily be missed if you do not know where to look for it, especially when you have been conditioned to clean your plate. Also, if you start eating when you are not hungry, it's hard to know when to stop out of fullness.

How do you *imagine* comfortable satiety feels? Here are some common descriptions offered by our clients:

- A subtle feeling of stomach fullness
- Feeling satisfied and content
- Nothingness—neither hungry nor full

The sensation is highly individual. And while we can describe it endlessly, it's akin to trying to tell someone what snow feels like.

We can give you a good idea—but it's something that needs to be experienced at the personal level, so that *you* know how it feels, in *your* body.

HOW TO RESPECT YOUR FULLNESS

When you habitually clean your plate, your eating style easily goes on autopilot—you eat until completion, until the food is gone. To break this pattern of eating, we have found it helpful to be keenly aware or hyperconscious of your eating. This means being conscious or mindful of your eating experience. While you may certainly be aware that you are engaged in the act of eating, we find that somewhere between bites one and one hundred there is a significant level of unconsciousness. Quite often the food is not even being tasted! Likewise, it's all too easy to bypass comfortable satiety. Here are some examples:

- I wasn't aware of how much candy I would eat at the movies until suddenly, my hands were scratching at the bottom of the empty box.
- I wouldn't even consider splitting a meal when eating out until my boss asked if I would split an entree at her favorite restaurant. Begrudgingly, I agreed. To my surprise I was thoroughly satisfied with half an entree, *knowing all too well that had I ordered the full portion I would have eaten it all, out of sheer habit.*
- Once I opened up a package of *any* food, I had to eat it all. God forbid I'd leave a few tidbits. I know I'm not even tasting the food most of the time.

Conscious Eating

The initial step away from the blind autopilot eating mode is *conscious eating*. It's a phase where you neutrally observe your eating as if under a microscope. (Your Food Anthropologist voice will be very helpful here.) We have broken this stage into a series of steps, which begins with taking a mini time-out from eating. This will help you regroup and assess where you are in your eating. It's like the time-out that athletes and coaches take during a game to help improve their play or strategy. Here's what to do.

- *Pause in the middle of a meal or snack for a time-out.* Keep in mind that this time-out is not a commitment to stop eating. Rather, it's a commitment to being in check with your body and taste buds. (If you thought that by pausing, you were obligated to leave food on your plate, you'd be reluctant to go through this step. In fact, many of our clients who initially appeared resistant to this step, later admitted that they were afraid that they would have to stop eating from that point on.) During this time-out, perform these checks:

TASTE CHECK: We find that this check is usually pleasurable, which is why we like to begin with it. Ask yourself how the food tastes. Is it worthy of your taste buds? Or are you continuing to eat just because the food is there?

SATIETY CHECK: Ask yourself what your hunger or fullness level is. Are you still hungry, do you feel unsatisfied, or is your hunger going away and are you beginning to feel satisfied? In the beginning, this may seem like a hit-or-miss process. Be patient, and remember, you are getting to know yourself from the inside out. Just as you would not expect to get to know a person over one meal, how could you expect to understand your satiety level in one meal or snack? It will take time. However, the more in tune you are with your hunger level, and the more you honor your hunger, the easier this step will be. Remember to be open to any answer. There can be considerable fluctuation in your fullness levels depending upon the last time you ate and what you ate. If you find you're still hungry, then resume eating.

- *When you finish eating* (whatever the amount), *ask yourself where your fullness level is now.* Did you reach comfortable satiety? Did you surpass it? By how much? Use the Fullness Discovery scale to help you get in touch. Note: This is the same scale as the Hunger Discovery Scale on p. 74—only now we're focussing on fullness.

- *Discovering your fullness level will help you identify your Last-Bite Threshold.* This is the endpoint. You know that the bite of food *in* your mouth is your last—finis! It may take you a long time

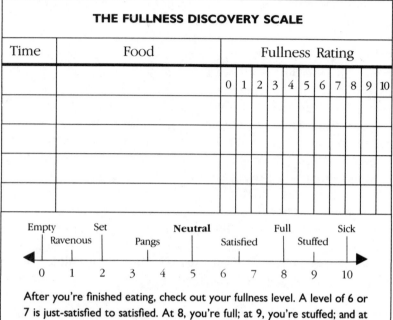

THE FULLNESS DISCOVERY SCALE

Time	Food	Fullness Rating										
		0	1	2	3	4	5	6	7	8	9	10

Empty   Set   **Neutral**   Full   Sick
　　Ravenous　　Pangs　　Satisfied　　Stuffed

◀　0　1　2　3　4　5　6　7　8　9　10　▶

After you're finished eating, check out your fullness level. A level of 6 or 7 is just-satisfied to satisfied. At 8, you're full; at 9, you're stuffed; and at 10, you are beginning to feel sick from overfilling. Work toward ending your eating at a 6 or 7. Ultimately, you'll find that the last-bite threshold corrolates with this level of satisfaction.

Remember, the hungrier you are when you begin eating, the higher your fullness number is likely to be when you stop. But, if you start eating at a 3 or a 4, you'll be more apt to stop at a 6 or 7—satisfied but not overfull.

to get to this point. The longer you have been disconnected from your body's sense of fullness, the longer it will take to identify this point. If you *honor your hunger* (Principle Two), it is much easier to know fullness. If however, you do not eat from biological hunger, how could you expect to stop from biological fullness (or to even know what it feels like)? Please be patient with yourself.

• *Don't feel obligated to leave food on your plate.* If you find that you have a level of resistance for this activity, it may be from past dieting experience. You may be feeling obligated to leave food on your plate—which is a remnant of the diet mentality. Remember, there is no commitment to leave food on your plate. The commitment, instead, is to getting to know your satiety level and your taste buds. It's perfectly normal, even when you discover your specific satiety level, to opt to overeat. That's okay. We have found that many clients continue to opt for more food—they are still testing the "unconditional permission" to eat. After a while, when the newness wears off, you will find that it's quite easy to leave food on your plate. It does require, however, a degree of consciousness—checking in with yourself. But if most of the time you can recognize your fullness, and respect it, it will make a considerable difference in your ability to maintain a natural weight.

How to Increase Consciousness

It's very difficult to do two conscious things at once. While you certainly may juggle a zillion activities, your mind focuses primarily on one. That's why, for example, so many people lock their keys in their car. Their minds are focused somewhere else, such as getting into the office on time, or unloading the groceries. We find that to get the most out of eating, it needs to be a conscious activity, whenever possible.

• *Eat Without Distraction.* Value and enjoy the eating experience when possible. For example, Adelle, a fast-paced, hard-driven lawyer, always made the best use of her time, and would usually eat while doing something else. Adelle would read briefs while eating lunch at work and would dine with a magazine at home. She took a step forward when she decided to try eating without distraction when at home (she was too busy at work to even consider "just eating" lunch). Adelle discovered that if she ate a meal or snack at home without engaging in reading, she would usually eat less. To her surprise, she learned that she ate less not because she was trying to eat smaller amounts, but because she could detect her fullness level much sooner. She was thrilled that "without trying" she was eating less food, feeling satisfied without deprivation, and not dieting. Adelle was willing to eat this way at home, but did not view it as realistic for work—and this was progress!

• *Reinforce Your Conscious Decision to Stop.* Many of our clients have found that when *they* decide to stop eating, because they've reached the last-bite threshold, it's helpful to *do* something to make it a conscious act, such as gently nudging the plate forward half an inch or putting their utensils or napkin on their plate. This simply reminds them of their decision. Otherwise, it may be all too easy to innocently nibble on the remaining food, even though you had no intention of doing so. (If you have trouble with the idea of wasting food, try putting your leftovers away for tomorrow's lunch or dinner or giving them to a homeless person.)

• *Defend Yourself from Obligatory Eating.* This usually means practicing saying, "No, thank you!" I never realized the significance of this act until I (ET) attended a very elegant cocktail party in which there seemed to be one waiter for each guest! The moment my hand was empty of food or drink, an all-too-eager waiter was there to offer more food or beverage. I found it was so much easier to say "yes," especially if I was in the middle of a conversation. It took much more energy to say "no." The same is true if you attend any function in which there are well-meaning "food-pushers," from the gracious host to the obnoxious relative. A special note of caution to those of you who enjoy wine by the bottle at a good restaurant: A good server will often keep your glass full. Unless you are conscious of that, you may drink more than you intend. Remember, *you* are in charge of how much to eat or drink.

THE FULLNESS FACTORS

"I just ate two hours ago—I honored my hunger *and* respected my fullness, so how could I be hungry again so soon?" While the ebb and tide of satiety signals may seem puzzling, it's quite normal to have different degrees of hunger and fullness, especially when you begin listening to your body's eating cues. There are also several factors that affect fullness. These factors are both biological and learned. When you have a general understanding of some of these satiety factors, it makes it easier to trust your body and *feel your fullness*.

The ability to recognize comfortable satiety or fullness can ultimately determine how much food will be consumed in a meal. And the amount of food eaten in a meal is influenced by these fullness factors:

• *The amount of time* that has passed since the last time you ate. The more often you eat, the less hungry you will be. This has been found to be true in nibbling studies. These are studies in which people are given several snacks or mini-meals throughout the day. The nibblers prove consistently *less* hungry than those fed identical calories divided into three larger meals. While the purpose of these studies has been to examine the metabolic effects of snacking compared to traditional meals, the researchers have consistently noted that the nibblers were less hungry, even though calories and fat offered were identical in both groups.

• *The kind of food you eat.* The macronutrients, protein, carbohydrates, and fat influence subsequent food intake by their contribution to the total amount of food energy in the stomach. Other food factors such as fiber will also affect the fullness factor because of its bulk and water-retention properties. Protein in particular seems to have a suppressive effect on intake beyond its contribution to total calories, according to several studies.

• *The amount of food still remaining in the stomach* at the time of eating. If your stomach is empty you will eat more than if some food is still present (from a prior snack or meal).

• *Initial hunger level.* If you begin a meal or snack in a famished state, you are more likely to overeat, and override satiety signals.

• *Social influence.* Eating with other people can influence how much *you* eat. Studies have shown that:
—The more people gathered at a meal, the more people tend to eat.
—Eating with others increases the duration of the meal.
—Eating more on weekends is usually due to being around people.
—Dieters, however, have been shown to eat less when they

know someone is "watching" them. The same is true for nondieters, when they dine with a "model" eater. In one study, when the model eater refrained from eating, so too did the nondieter.

There is a tendency to ignore or be distracted from biological signals in social settings. We have found that the key to the social dilemma is to continue making eating a *conscious* activity with purposeful food choices.

Clearly, there are many factors that influence how full you feel from eating. With so many variables that exert influence on your eating, it should be no surprise then, that the amount of food you desire to eat can and will fluctuate. A big key is to stay tuned in and to eat consciously.

Beware of Air Food

Simply shoving some food in your mouth like a pacifier to ease hunger pangs may backfire, and the comforting effect may not be long-lasting. This is especially true of "*air food*"—food that fills up the stomach but offers little sustenance. Air food includes such low-calorie foods as air-popped popcorn, rice cakes, puffed rice cereal, fat-free crackers, celery sticks, and calorie-free beverages. There's nothing inherently wrong with these foods. But if you eat them expecting to get full, it will often take massive quantities—and you might find yourself on the prowl for something more substantial to "top off the meal." That's where having a balanced snack or meal, which includes a heavier carbohydrate, some protein, or a little fat, is especially helpful, if you're looking for a little "staying power," or the stick-to-your-ribs kind of feeling from eating.

If, on the other hand, you know you will be going out for a fabulous dinner or to a party, and want just a little something to take the edge off your hunger, lighter foods may serve your purpose just fine.

Foods with Staying Power

Snacks or meals with a little fiber, complex carbohydrates, some protein, or even a little fat will help increase satiety. Ironically, many of our chronic dieters shy away from the very foods that could help them feel more satisfied at meals—complex carbohydrates. Here are some common unsatisfying food choices and suggestions for how you can round them out to be more satisfying. (There's nothing inherently wrong with these light foods, they just may not provide staying power.)

Less Filling Foods:	Staying Power Boost: Add these types of foods to perk up your satiety
Salad (no carbohydrates; little protein unless it's an entree)	Protein: tuna, chicken, garbanzo or kidney beans
	Carbs: Crackers, whole grain roll
Fresh fruit (no protein; can be low on carbs depending on quantity)	Protein/Carb: lowfat cheese and whole grain crackers; half sandwich; nonfat yogurt
Turkey breast (no fiber, no carbs)	Carb: whole grain pita; whole grain bagel; whole grain crackers

WHAT IF YOU CAN'T STOP EATING?

If you discover after time that you still are eating even though you are not hungry, there's a good chance that you might be using food as a coping mechanism. This is not always as obvious and dramatic as some magazines suggest. Chapter 11 is devoted to this issue.

WHAT IF YOU FEEL THERE'S SOMETHING MISSING?

If you've discovered what it feels like to feel comfortably full, and yet feel that something is missing, it could be the satisfaction factor. This is so important we've devoted a whole principle to it—and discuss it in the next chapter.

Chapter Ten

PRINCIPLE 6:

Discover the Satisfaction Factor

The Japanese have the wisdom to promote pleasure as one of their goals of healthy living. In our fury to be thin and healthy, we often overlook one of the most basic gifts of existence—the pleasure and satisfaction that can be found in the eating experience. When you eat what you really want, in an environment that is inviting, the pleasure you derive will be a powerful force in helping you feel satisfied and content. By providing this experience for yourself, you will find that it takes much less food to decide you've had "enough."

How many times have you eaten a rice cake when you really wanted potato chips? And how many rice cakes, carrots, and apples have you eaten attempting to get the same satisfaction you would have found with a handful of chips? If you feel truly satisfied with your eating experience, you will find that you eat far less food. Conversely, if you are unsatisfied, you will likely eat more and be on the prowl, regardless of your satiety level.

For example, one client, Fran, wanted a piece of cornbread with lunch, but she fastidiously refrained from eating it. Fran thought about having cornbread with dinner, but again stopped herself. That night, she ate six Weight Watchers desserts, and realized that what she was really seeking was cornbread—no amount of diet desserts would satisfy her cornbread craving. Ironically, the calories from the diet desserts far exceeded the calories from a single piece of cornbread. When Fran was eating the diet desserts, she was chasing her *phantom food*—trying to fill the void created by denying the satisfaction factor from the food she originally wanted.

THE WISDOM OF PLEASURE

Americans have gotten so focused on the alchemy of foods—whether as an adjunct to losing weight or seeking health—that we have neglected a very important role that eating plays in our lives—provision of pleasure. The Japanese promote pleasure as one of their goals of healthy eating. *"Make all activities pertaining to food and eating pleasurable ones,"* is one of their *Dietary Guidelines for Health Promotion.* How ironic this advice is for Americans, especially dieters, who have come to see food as the enemy and the eating experience as the battleground between "tempting" foods and the willpower to avoid them. Most dieters with whom we work have lost sight of how important it is to have a satisfying, let alone pleasurable, eating experience. For some, any experience that smacks of pleasure triggers feelings of guilt and wrongdoing. It's not too surprising, since we live in a society with strong Puritanical roots and a tradition of self-denial. Dieting plays right in to this ethic—make sacrifices, settle for less. Yet if you settle for food that is inferior, it will often leave you wanting . . . eating . . . overeating.

Jill is an example of a young woman who let the fear of eating pleasurable foods turn her into a restrictive eater. Her food choices were based primarily on their weight-reducing powers. She was convinced that if she even tasted a pleasurable food, she would never again be able to control herself. Every time that Jill was in a dieting phase, she would find herself having strong cravings for forbidden foods. She chased her "phantom food," searching for a food that would quell her cravings. If she craved a chocolate cookie, she would spread sugar-free jam on fat-free saltines. When that didn't satisfy her, she'd go on to cinnamon-flavored rice cakes, then to fat-free "healthy" cookies (which she disliked and "tasted like sweetened cardboard") and lots of dried fruit. By the end of an evening, *Jill would have eaten ten times more calories in her diet foods than she would have eaten had she just allowed herself to have the chocolate cookie.* And, not surprisingly, she would usually "succumb" to the chocolate cookie anyway at the end of her frustrating food chase.

After learning the Intuitive Eating process, Jill quit her phantom food searches and allowed herself to eat what she really wanted. She can now even order a hamburger with fries and find that she ends up leaving half of her food because she's so *satisfied*. She's also found that it isn't often she actually even wants to eat those kinds of foods!

DON'T BE AFRAID TO ENJOY YOUR FOOD

Like Jill, our clients are initially afraid that if they let the pleasure of eating into their lives, they might continue to seek food in an uncontrollable fashion. Yet, letting yourself enjoy food will actually result in self-limiting, rather than out-of-control eating. Remember, as we explained in Chapter 7, deprivation is a key factor that leads to backlash eating.

Satisfied Now—Eat Less Later

For many of our clients, feeling a sense of satisfaction in a meal actually decreases their yearning for foods at a later time. We have had our clients compare having a full-course meal for dinner with just "picking" or scrounging. When they take the time to prepare a meal that attracts their sense of smell, taste, sight, and so forth, they invariably report a feeling of satisfaction and a decreased need for more food later in the evening. Those who come home and drop on the sofa with a box of crackers and a soda find themselves getting up at each commercial for yet another snack. They feel that they haven't really eaten and never seem to be satisfied. By the end of the evening, they feel overfull and frustrated.

Kelly is a busy person who often neglects her own needs. Sometimes she'll be so busy with work and her child that she doesn't stop to prepare an entire meal for herself. On the days when she takes the time to figure out what she really wants to eat and ends up eating exactly what she wants for lunch or dinner, she finds that she has no desire for dessert. On the days when she diets all day and never feels satisfied, her dessert cravings at night are insatiable.

When you allow yourself pleasure and satisfaction from every possible eating experience, your total quantity of food will decrease.

HOW TO REGAIN YOUR
PLEASURE IN EATING

As a result of dieting, and the fear of giving it up, dieters have lost their pleasure in eating and they don't know how to get it back. Here are the steps we use with our clients to help them achieve pleasure and satisfaction in their eating.

STEP I:
ASK YOURSELF WHAT YOU *REALLY* WANT TO EAT

Satisfaction is derived when you take the time to figure out what you really want to eat, give yourself unconditional permission to eat it, and then eat in a relaxing enjoyable atmosphere.

The problem for most dieters with whom we've worked is that they have figured out so many "tricks" to avoid eating that they no longer know what they like to eat! When you're about to begin a new diet, have you ever asked yourself what you *feel like* eating? That thought rarely enters a dieter's mind. After all, the basic premise of dieting is to be told what to eat—why would you begin to question your own needs!

Such was the case with a forty-year-old woman, Jennifer, who had been overweight and dieting all of her life. As a child she was put on diets by her mother and her doctors. When Jennifer first visited my (ER) office, she belligerently stated that she didn't want to hear another word about dieting. She had only come because her doctor had insisted, and she emphatically stated that she knew everything there was to know about dieting. I told her that I didn't believe in dieting, and that all I really wanted to know was what she liked to eat. Astonishment crossed her face. She could hardly respond, but when she did, she told me that no one in her entire life had ever asked her what *she* wanted to eat. She had been on diets since she was a child and had always been told what she *should* eat. She went deep into thought for a few moments and then said that she had no idea what she liked. In fact, this morbidly obese woman wasn't even sure if she liked food at all.

At the end of the session, I suggested that Jennifer spend the next week experimenting with food so she could learn more about her taste preferences. During that week, Jennifer could only find ten foods that she actually liked, and discovered that she could do without the rest! The following week, Jennifer's task was to eat only those ten foods and see how much she actually consumed. Again, she was surprised by the results. When she ate what she liked, she found that she was satisfied by much less and that her total food intake that week was lower than it had been in years. One night, all she had for dinner was a scoop of chocolate ice cream. In the past she would down a huge dinner of foods she thought she should eat and would then finish the half-gallon of ice cream, because she felt guilty about having any of it!

Jennifer was on her way to becoming an Intuitive Eater. In addition to appreciating that she could have exactly what she wanted any time that she ate, she realized that eating when she was hungry would give her the most satisfaction. As a result of this revelation, she found herself eating only when she was hungry. She also found that eating past comfortable fullness was pointless, as the food no longer tasted good and her body felt miserable. Soon it became automatic for her to eat smaller quantities than she ever had in her life. Since she felt good for the first time in her life, she was motivated to begin a program of regular swimming—not because she *had to* but because she *wanted to* feel even better physically. Her obesity had led to problems with her knees and virtual inactivity. Jennifer went on to lose fifty pounds from the changes in her eating style, combined with her newfound physical activity. She felt continually satisfied by her meals, without feeling deprived.

If you also have trouble figuring out what you truly like to eat, the next step will give you clarification.

STEP 2:
DISCOVER THE PLEASURES OF THE PALATE

Our clients are focused on every aspect of food except the here and now. They lament the past and worry about the future (what will I eat, how will I work off these calories), but very rarely do they focus on the actual experience of eating. Therefore, they are not tasting— not experiencing or savoring food. It's almost as if the art of eating needs to be relearned without bias.

The Sensual Qualities of Foods

To discover what foods you really like, and how to increase satisfaction in your eating, explore the sensual qualities of foods. For most people, this means a conscious period of experimentation. Take your taste buds and palate for a sensory joy ride. Before you eat, consider:

• *Taste.* Put a particular food in your mouth to see which of your taste sensations gets stimulated. Roll the food around on your tongue to see if it's predominantly sweet, salty, sour, or bitter. Is that taste pleasant, neutral, or maybe even offensive? Try this experiment at various times during the day to see if certain tastes are more pleasurable at different times. Some people are drawn to the sweet taste at breakfast and want waffles or pancakes. Something spicy, such as eggs with salsa, might be a turn-off early in the morning. Others can't think of something sweet until later in the afternoon.

• *Texture.* As you roll the food around on your tongue and begin to chew on it, experience the various types of textures that foods can provide. How does crunchy feel to you? Is it abrasive to have to break into a crunchy food, or is it a satisfying experience? What reaction do you have to a food that is smooth or creamy? Does it remind you of baby food, and is that appealing or annoying? Some foods are chewy and require a lot of work by your teeth and tongue. What is that like for you? Sometimes you might just want the flow of a liquid through your mouth and down your throat. Certain food textures might be appealing at different times of the day, or even on different days.

• *Aroma.* Sometimes the aroma of a food will have more of an effect on your desire for it than does its taste or texture. Appreciate the various aromas that foods can emit. Walk by the bakery and smell the yeasty bread coming out of the oven, or inhale the coffee vapors as the coffee is dripping through the filter. If the aroma of a food is not appealing, you probably won't get your optimal satisfaction from it. If it smells great to you as it is cooking or served to you, however, it will probably increase your satisfaction.

• *Appearance.* Food artists who design commercial food sets or menus for restaurants know that foods that look appealing are alluring and make a person want to try them. Take a look at the food you're about to eat. Is it attractive to your eye? Is it fresh looking? Is its color interesting to you? Imagine a plate with a poached chicken breast, a boiled potato, and cauliflower—not too thrilling. You'll probably get less satisfaction from that meal than one that's more exciting to look at.

• *Temperature.* A steamy bowl of soup might just be the order of the day if it's cold and rainy outside. But chilly frozen yogurt is not usually desirable when you're shivering under an umbrella. Ask yourself what is the most appealing temperature of your foods. Do you like your hot foods boiling hot or temperate? Do you like your cold drinks with lots of ice or very little? Or is room temperature just fine for you for everything?

• *Volume or Filling-Capacity.* Some foods are light and airy, while others are heavy and filling. The filling capacity of your food choices can make a difference in how much food you need to satisfy you or how you feel after you're finished eating. Some days you might only be satisfied by a plate of pasta which fills your stomach, while at other times, a lighter salad is more appealing. Even if something tastes and feels great on your tongue and in your mouth, if it makes your stomach feel queasy or too heavy it will diminish the satisfying experience.

Respect Your Individual Taste Buds. Keep in mind that everyone has a different experience with taste and texture sensations. Not all foods will be desirable to you. (If you once got sick on corn, regardless of the cause, corn might never seem appealing again.) Your preferences may be lifelong or may change from time to time. Keep in touch with what is appetizing to you so that you can choose what is most satisfying.

Think About What You Really Feel Like Eating

Once you've gone through this hyperconscious experimentation with the sensory qualities of foods, the next time you feel like a meal or a snack, take a few moments to decide what you *really* want to eat. If you have trouble deciding what to eat, or need a little clarity, ask yourself:

- What do I feel like eating?
- What food aroma might appeal to me?
- How will the food look to my eye?
- How will the food taste and feel in my mouth?
- Do I want something sweet, salty, sour, or even slightly bitter?
- Do I want something crunchy, smooth, creamy, soft, lumpy, fluid, etc?
- Do I want something hot, cold, or moderate?
- Do I want something light, airy, heavy, filling, or in between?
- How will my stomach feel when I'm finished eating?

If you have a general knowledge of your taste preferences, it will lead you to the right place on the menu or in the supermarket. Checking in with yourself before a meal will give you the specifics of the moment.

A further critical key to finding satisfaction in your eating is to take a time-out *after* you've had a few bites of your food. Is the taste and texture consistent with your desire? Is the food satisfying enough to eat? If you continue to eat a food just because it's there, despite the fact that it's unappealing, you'll only end up feeling unsatisfied when you're finished and find yourself on the prowl for something else that will satisfy you.

STEP 3:
MAKE YOUR EATING EXPERIENCE MORE ENJOYABLE

Savor Your Food

Europeans seem to have cornered the market on slow, sensual eating experiences. Businesses often shut down temporarily to allow for a long lingering lunch, so the meal can be savored and appreciated. Friends tend to gather together to enjoy the conversation and the food. Americans, on the other hand, often engage in desktop dining (fifteen minutes if they're lucky) while going over notes for a meeting. Who do you think has the most satisfying meal experience?

Alice is an executive in a company that stresses high productivity.

Taking time to sit down for lunch is unheard of, and she's so anxious to get into the office in the morning to begin her calls to the East Coast that she never allows herself to eat breakfast at home before she leaves. By the time Alice gets home in the evening, the frenetic pace of her day has become a part of her—she ends up gulping down her entire dinner before her husband and daughter get through their salads.

When you race through your meals as Alice does, you don't give yourself the opportunity to experience the sensual aspects of your food. You don't have time to appreciate the attractiveness of the different colors and shapes of the food. You can barely take in their aromas or feel their textures on your tongue and teeth—let alone savor their taste.

To help you savor your food and get more satisfaction from your meals:

- Make time to appreciate your food. Give yourself a distinct time allowance for a meal. Even fifteen minutes is better than nothing.
- Sit down at the table or your desk. Standing at the refrigerator or walking around decreases attention and satisfaction.
- Take several deep breaths before you begin to eat. Deep breathing helps to calm and center you, so you can be focused on eating slowly.
- Pay attention to eating as slowly as you can. Remember that your taste buds are on your tongue, not in your stomach. Gobbling your food takes away your chance to really taste it.
- Taste each bite of food that you put in your mouth. Experience the different taste and texture sensations the food can provide.
- Put your fork down now and then throughout the meal. This will help to slow you down.
- Remember Principle Five: *Respect Your Fullness*. Take a time-out in the midst of the meal to check your fullness level (see Chapter 9). Food won't taste as good or be as satisfying after you've reached the last-bite threshold.

Eat When Gently Hungry Rather
Than When Overhungry

If you sit down for a meal when you're so hungry that you could eat a cow, you won't be able to tell the difference between a delicious steak and the cow itself! If you're overhungry, your biological need for energy supersedes your ability to eat slowly and taste what's before you. Likewise, if you begin to eat when you aren't really hungry, it can be difficult to decide whether what you're eating is really what you want and whether it's satisfying. When you're not very hungry, food is not as compelling. If you find this is true for you, this may be a sign that you're not ready to eat just yet. Wait a little while, until your hunger is somewhat more obvious, and you'll find that you'll have an easier time getting in touch with what you really want to eat.

Eat in a Pleasant Environment (When Possible)

Most people find that they get the greatest satisfaction from their meals by eating them in a pleasing setting. Restaurants spend a great deal of time and money creating an environment that is appealing and will draw people back again and again. The aesthetics of a restaurant can be as important as the taste of the food. At home, the same thing goes. If you set your table in a pleasing manner (a placemat or tablecloth, pretty china, and so forth), your food enjoyment will increase. But eating while standing or driving can diminish satisfaction. If you eat in the car, you are distracted by the traffic and by having to balance food on your lap.

Avoid Tension

Keep heated fights off-limits at the table. One of the surest ways to decrease your satisfaction in eating is to try to eat when you're having an argument with a family member or friend. You'll probably end up eating faster and might even use your chewing as a way to show your anger. You definitely won't have your focus on the food and might eat everything before you without even noticing it—not a satisfying experience!

Provide Variety

Eating a variety of foods is not only nutritionally wise, but it will give you a much broader and more satisfying eating experience. Many of our clients take pride in keeping empty refrigerators and barren cupboards. They believe that if certain foods aren't around, they'll be less tempted to overeat. The reality is that a lack of appealing food choices creates a sense of deprivation and promotes a creative food-foraging experience that never seems to produce a satisfying result. Give yourself the gift of keeping a variety of foods around, from soups to pastas to cookies or fruits and vegetables. You never know what you might feel like eating. Finding satisfaction in your eating will be a futile attempt if what you want isn't there.

STEP 4:
DON'T SETTLE

You are not obligated to finish eating a food just because you took a bite of it. Yet how often have you tasted what appeared to be a mouth-watering dessert, only to discover it was mediocre—and yet you kept on eating? One of the biggest assets of being an Intuitive Eater is the ability to toss aside food that isn't to your liking. This can be easily done when you are truly tasting and experiencing food, combined with the knowledge you can eat whatever you want again.

For the most part, adopt the motto: *"If you don't love it, don't eat it, and if you love it, savor it."* Order something else, find something different in the refrigerator, or eat the parts of the meal that you like and leave the rest. For example, Barbara spoke of a meal served to her at a banquet that was comprised of salad, chicken, vegetables, and pasta. She took just one taste of the salad and left the rest when she found that the lettuce was soggy under a sea of dressing that she didn't like. The chicken and pasta were delicious, so she ate most of them. The vegetables were so buttery that they overwhelmed her taste buds, so she left them on the plate. In her old diet days, she would have eaten only the salad and vegetables, thinking that was the "diet" way to do it, and she would have left her meal unsatisfied, only to go home in search of something else to eat.

Melody is another client who is learning to discard what she doesn't find satisfying. One of Melody's favorite foods is a trademark muffin at a local restaurant. Every time she goes to the restaurant, she savors her muffin and feels satisfied. One day, Melody got the inspired notion to bake the trademark muffins from the restaurant's prepared mix. And bake she did. When she took a bite of a freshly baked muffin, she was sadly disappointed. It didn't taste anything like what she had eaten in the restaurant. Melody's connection with her Intuitive Eating allowed her to throw out the muffins, with the conviction that she would only eat them when she could get the "real thing."

STEP 5:
CHECK IN: DOES IT STILL TASTE GOOD?

Have you ever eaten a whole bag of cookies or a whole carton of Häagan-Dazs? If so, you can probably attest to the fact that the first couple of cookies or spoonsful of ice cream tasted much better than those at the bottom of the barrel. Even the taste satisfaction of a large apple dwindles by the time you get down to the core. In studies of hedonics to food cues (hedonics is the branch of psychology dealing with pleasurable and unpleasurable feelings), researchers find that continued exposure to the same food results in a decrease of desire for that food. We also see that in our clients.

Try your own hedonic experiment. Rate the taste pleasure you get from the first few bites of a food from one to ten—one being the least pleasurable and ten being the most. Then stop halfway through eating the food and check your taste buds. Finally, rate the food when you're down to the last bite. You're likely to find that the numbers diminish along with the food.

Routinely, check in with yourself to see if the food tastes as good as it did when you started. If it doesn't, consider stopping, as your satisfaction level is diminishing by the biteful. Wait until you're hungry again. Food will taste better and you'll be more satisfied. And, remember, no one is going to take that food away from your eating repertoire. You can have it for the rest of your life. So why waste your time and your food on a less than satisfying experience!

IT DOESN'T HAVE TO BE PERFECT

We've discussed how taking the time to figure out what you really want to eat, and eating in a favorable environment, can lead you to more pleasurable, satisfying eating experiences. But what if this isn't always possible? There will be times when you don't have the option of getting exactly what you want. You might be served a meal at a friend's or relative's house that has little to say for it. Many a client has bemoaned meals made by a mother-in-law or an old friend who might boil the vegetables until unrecognizable or cook the chicken until it's the texture of an old shoe. At those times, remember the principle of thinking in gray rather than in black and white (see Chapter 8). Intuitive Eating is not a process that seeks perfection, but one that offers guidelines to a comfortable relationship with food. Remember, most of your eating experiences will be more satisfying and pleasurable than you've experienced in years of diets. It's only one meal—you will survive. It's how you jump back into taking care of yourself afterward that makes the difference.

Sometimes *honoring your hunger* is the best you can do. And for many of our patients, that alone is significant progress. But if survival eating occupies most of your experiences with food, your satisfaction factor will most likely be low.

RECLAIM YOUR RIGHT TO PLEASURABLE, SATISFYING EATING

If dieting has been a significant part of your life for many years, you may need to make a serious effort to reclaim your right to enjoy your food. You may have been so programmed to eat what you were told, especially foods that have little taste pleasure, that you hardly know where to begin to find satisfaction. *Knowing what you like to eat, and believing that you have the right to enjoy food, are key factors in a lifetime of weight control without dieting.* If it takes you some time to accomplish all of this, be patient. After all, it's taken you many years to lose your ability to truly enjoy eating.

Chapter Eleven

PRINCIPLE 7:

Cope with Your Emotions Without Using Food

Find ways to comfort, nurture, distract, and resolve your issues without using food. Anxiety, loneliness, boredom, and anger are emotions we all experience throughout life. Each has its own trigger, and each has its own appeasement. Food won't fix any of these feelings. It may comfort for the short term, distract from the pain, or even numb you into a food hangover. But food won't solve the problem. If anything, eating for an emotional hunger will only make you feel worse in the long run. You'll ultimately have to deal with the source of the emotion, as well as the discomfort of overeating.

Eating doesn't occur in a void. Regardless of your weight, food usually has emotional associations. If you have any doubt, catch a glimpse of food commercials. They push our eating buttons—not through our stomachs but through the emotional connection. They imply that in sixty seconds or less you can:

- Capture romance with an intimate cup of coffee.
- Bake someone happy.
- Reward yourself with a rich dessert.

Eating can be one of the most emotionally laden experiences that we have in our lives. The emotional rhythm to eating is set from the first day that the infant is offered the breast or the bottle to quell his crying. It's then reinforced each time a cookie is offered to soothe a scraped knee, or ice cream is eaten to celebrate a Little League victory. Nearly every culture and religion uses food as an important symbolic custom, from the American Thanksgiving feast to the Jewish Passover seder. Each time a significant life experience is celebrated with food, the emotional connection deepens, from the I-got-the-promotion dinner celebration to the annual birthday cake. Likewise, each time food is used for a little wound-licking or comfort, the emotional bond strengthens.

Food is love, food is comfort, food is reward, food is a reliable friend. And, sometimes, food becomes your *only* friend in moments of pain and loneliness.

Our patients are embarrassed that food can become so important—that food is their best friend. But if you consider how emotionally charged food is, it's no surprise that food can evolve into a special salvo. When a dieter overeats during rough emotional times (whether periodically or chronically), it is usually obvious that food is used as a coping mechanism. For other dieters, it is not so clear.

Some of our clients are emotionally unaware—they have not yet learned to identify their feelings. It may not be obvious to them that they are using food to cope. Sometimes, these clients don't know why they are eating. Often the "why" is an uncomfortable feeling that has not been discovered. Or they may be engaged in a subtle form of emotional eating, such as boredom eating. Nibbling to kill time between classes or appointments is not emotionally charged, but the results can be the same as using food to numb strong feelings—*overeating.*

The eating experience itself, especially overeating, evokes feelings, and those feelings can affect your ability to eat normally. One of the most detrimental feelings that overeating can stir up is guilt and shame. Studies have shown that although you might have immediate emotional comfort from eating, the negative rush of guilt that bursts forth is powerful enough to completely wipe out the relief.

Becoming an Intuitive Eater means learning to be gentle with yourself about how you use food to cope, and letting go of the guilt. As odd as this may sound, eating may have been the only mechanism you had to get through difficult times in your life. It may also have been an inevitable result of years of dieting and feelings of deprivation and despair that arose from dieting. *Dieting itself can trigger emotions which ultimately lead to using food to cope with these feelings*—chalk up another vicious cycle caused by dieting.

THE CONTINUUM OF EMOTIONAL EATING

Food can be used to cope with feelings in a myriad of ways. Using food in this way is not a component of biological hunger, but of emotional hunger. Emotional eating is triggered by feelings, such as boredom or anger, not by hunger. These feelings can trigger anything from a benign nibble to an out-of-control binge.

It's important to understand that this coping mechanism lies on a continuum of intensity that begins at one end with mild, almost universal sensory eating to the opposite end with numbing, often anesthetizing eating. The following diagram illustrates this spectrum:

sensory
gratification • comfort • distraction • sedation • punishment

◄──►

Sensory Gratification

The mildest, and most common feeling that food can call forth is pleasure. The significance of receiving pleasure from eating is emphasized in Principle Six: *Discover the Satisfaction Factor*. This concept is not only critical to Intuitive Eating, but is a normal, natural part of living. Don't underestimate the importance of pleasing your palate. As we explained in Chapter 10, by letting yourself enjoy and appreciate eating, you will actually reduce the amount of food you need to feel satisfied when biologically hungry. For example, allowing yourself little tastes of the special foods available at Thanksgiving will usually offset overeating.

Comfort

Just the thought of certain foods has the ability to evoke feelings from a comfortable time or place. For example, do you ever crave chicken soup when you are sick or macaroni and cheese on dreary days—because that's what your mom fixed on these occasions? Those are examples of comfort foods. It's normal to have a repertoire of comfort foods. If you want to curl up with a blanket in front of a fireplace and sip hot cocoa with your dinner, that's fine. Eating comfort foods occasionally can be part of a healthy relationship with food, if you do it while staying in touch with your satiety levels and without guilt. If, however, food is the first and only thing that comes to mind to take care of you when you are feeling sad, lonely, or uncomfortable, it can become a destructive coping mechanism.

Distraction

If you go a little further on the continuum of emotional eating, food can be used to distract you from feelings you choose not to experience. Using food to cope in this way can become troublesome, as it can be a seductive behavior that blocks your ability to detect your intuitive signals. It also can inhibit you from discovering the source of the feelings and taking care of your true needs. Whether you're the teenager who sits in front of the TV with a bag of chips to distract you from the feelings of boredom in doing your home-work, or you're an executive who goes through a whole bowl of peanuts on your desk to distract you from the anxiety of an arduous meeting, this kind of eating needs to be confronted. There is nothing wrong with occasionally wanting to distract yourself from feelings. Experiencing your feelings twenty-four hours a day can be tedious and overwhelming. *But food is not an appropriate distractor for temporary relief.* (Alternative distractors are mentioned later in the chapter.)

Sedation

A more serious form of using food to cope is eating for the purpose of numbing or anesthetizing. One client calls this form of eating a "food coma." Another suggests that this kind of eating results in a "food hangover." In either case, eating to sedate yourself can be as emotionally dangerous as using drugs or alcohol for this purpose. It keeps you from experiencing any feeling for extended periods of time. It becomes impossible to sense your intuitive signals of hunger and satiety, and it deprives you of the satisfying experience that food can bring to your life. Most clients who use food in this way talk about feeling out of control, out of touch with life, and generally zoned-out. They also have trouble recognizing basic sensations of hunger and fullness.

Connie is a young woman who had an abusive childhood. She learned to use food at a very early age as a numbing agent. She continues to sedate herself through the anxiety, fear, and sadness of her present life. Connie's weight can escalate five pounds a week when she is regularly going into her "food comas." But even more frightening than her weight gain is the complete detachment from life that she experiences each time. She isolates herself from her friends, calls in sick to work, and feels completely hopeless about life itself. Connie is learning to utilize other coping tools so that she can improve the quality of her life.

When eating to numb and sedate is occasional and short term, it tends to have little detrimental effect. But this kind of eating can escalate into an addictive behavior before you even notice it.

Punishment

Sometimes, eating for the purpose of sedation becomes so frequent and intense that self-blame ensues and ultimately triggers punishing behaviors. Clients find themselves eating large quantities of food in an angry, forceful manner that allows them to feel beaten up. This is the most severe form of emotional eating and can lead to loss of self-esteem and to self-hatred. Clients who use food to punish themselves report no pleasure in their eating and actually begin to hate food. Fortunately, this type of eating behavior disappears when the Nurturer voice can be beckoned to give understanding and compassion. If there's no crime committed, no punishment need be tendered.

EMOTIONAL TRIGGERS

We've looked at general emotional reasons for eating; now let's examine the specific feelings involved. A craving for certain foods, or simply a desire to eat can be triggered by a variety of feelings and situations.

Some people use food to cope when they have no idea that's what they're doing. They think that they're overeating "just because it tastes good." If you find that you're doing quite a bit of eating when you're not biologically hungry, then there's a good chance that you are using food to cope. You may not have deep-seated emotional reasons for eating, but just getting through life's hassles with some of its irksome tasks and boredom might trigger you to seek food to make it all easier.

Boredom and Procrastination

One of the most common reasons our clients eat when they're not hungry is boredom. In fact, studies have shown that regardless of a person's weight, boredom is one of the most common triggers of emotional eating. One particular study divided college students into two groups. One group had the monotonous task of writing the same letters over and over again for nearly half an hour. The other group was engaged in a stimulating writing project. Students in each group were given a bowl of crackers to nibble on. Guess which group ate more? Regardless of weight, the "bored" group ate the most crackers.

In boredom eating, food is used as a way to fill time as well as a way to put off doing mundane work. For some people, the thought of the food and the actual experience of going for it and eating it breaks the tedium. Here are some situations that produce boredom eating.

- Lying around the house on a Sunday afternoon when you've made no plans for the day.
- Having to get through an afternoon of studying, paperwork, or a writing project.
- Watching a boring night of television with nothing else to do but take food breaks.
- Killing time: waiting for a meeting to get started, waiting for a phone call, and so forth. We also see this type of eating in our overworked clients—they feel they must always be *doing* something, being productive. The moment a tiny hole opens up in their schedule, they feel the need to fill it—often with food. (It's acceptable to eat, but not to rest!)

Bribery and Reward

Have you ever promised yourself that you could have a treat once you finished writing a term paper or a contract, or cleaning the house? If so, you have experienced reward eating. It's not unusual to use food as a motivation for accomplishing undesired tasks. For example:

- Children are often bribed with treats such as candy or ice cream if they behave—at the mall, for a babysitter, and so on.
- People often reward themselves for working hard: at work, at home, or at school with an extra bagel or a muffin, for example.

Using food as a reward can be self-perpetuating, as there will always be ongoing tasks and challenges which can be made more tolerable if they're mitigated by food gifts.

Excitement

Food and the eating experience itself can serve as a way to add excitement when life begins to feel dull. At a subtle level, planning a special meal or making a reservation at a favorite restaurant can create a sense of excitement.

The notion of going on a diet can trigger feelings of hope. This is one of the reasons why dieting is so alluring. Our clients talk of how even contemplating a new diet gives them a rush of adrenaline—just imagining a new body and a new life. When the diet fails, the excitement is replaced with despair. At this point, the experience of going to the store to buy large quantities of forbidden foods can be one way to recreate the excitement. And then the cycle continues—diet/overeating, diet/overeating. This is exciting, but at what cost?

Soothing

It's not hard to understand the soothing power that food can provide. It can be more appealing to go to the kitchen for cookies and milk than to sit on the couch and experience uncomfortable feelings. This is especially true if those cookies and milk remind you of a time that was pleasant and life felt less complicated. Habitually eating to soothe what ails you can evolve into a problem with food.

Food can have other symbolic associations with comfort. Ellen is a sixteen-year-old who has battled with her father since she was a small child. She describes him as mean and nasty with a bitter personality. It was not surprising to hear Ellen talk about her obsession with eating large amounts of candy every day as a way to bring "sweetness" into her life. To her, the sweets countered the bitterness of her daily experiences with her father.

Love

Food can become connected to the feeling of being loved. There is certainly a romantic link with food—chocolate on Valentine's Day is a classic example. When dating, there's an unspoken ground rule that your relationship is elevated to a more intimate level when you have experienced a home-cooked meal for two.

Clients frequently tell of how their parents' only way to show love was through food. These parents may not have been able to show physical attention or speak to them in loving ways, but food was always plentiful.

Frustration, Anger, and Rage

If you find yourself going through a bag of hard and crunchy pretzels when you're not hungry, it's a good bet that you may be feeling frustrated or angry. The physical act of biting and crunching can serve as a way to release these feelings for some people. One client, Nancy, a lawyer, discovered that she had a habit of subduing her anger at some of her clients by grabbing some hard food, whether it was carrots or crackers, and munching away.

Stress

Many of our clients say they head for the nearest candy bar under stressful times. Yet, in most individuals, biological mechanisms associated with stress *turn off* the desire to eat.

The rush of adrenaline during stressful times sets in motion a cascade of biological events to provide immediate energy. As a result, blood sugar is elevated and digestion is slowed. These two elements alone tend to suppress hunger and heighten the sense of satiety when eating. The biological reactions are a form of self-preservation—to ready our bodies for *"fight or flight."* While this was quite useful for survival—*fighting off* a man-eating tiger or *fleeing* from danger required immediate energy—a growing body of research suggests that in our modern day this mechanism may actually contribute to obesity. It may be stressful to *fight off* rush-hour traffic or to *flee* from a deadline, but you don't need the extra blood sugar that the stress reaction provides. Where does it go? If you don't use it (in the way of physical activity), excess blood sugar gets converted to fat. This biological problem is only compounded if you cope with stress by eating. Studies have also shown that people who have been dieting are especially vulnerable to overeating during stressful times. Stress becomes one more reason to "blow" the diet. Dieting itself can also be a source of stress.

Anxiety

Worries of any magnitude, from an upcoming final to waiting to hear if you got the job, can trigger an urgent need to eat to relieve anxiety. Sometimes generalized anxiety can be described as that uncomfortable feeling you are unable to put a finger on; our clients say it feels like butterflies in your stomach. With the focus on the stomach so goes the food.

Mild Depression

It's not uncommon for many people to turn to food when they are mildly depressed. In mild depression weight gain is often seen, especially in dieters. In one study, 62 percent of the dieters and 52 percent of nondieters stated they ate more when feeling depressed.

Being Connected

The need to feel part of a group or to feel a connection to others can be very powerful for some people, and can even affect how and what they eat. This experience was poignantly described by Mathew, when he was talking about the dinner he had eaten one night with some friends. Although he didn't like the food served, he ate it anyway. He made the choice to feel connected but dissatisfied with the food rather than feeling different. How many times have you eaten to be part of the crowd—from running out to get ice cream to sharing a pizza?

Loosening the Reins

Frequently, clients who are highly successful in every aspect of their lives, except in their eating, discount their accomplishments. They feel as if their food problems indicate they are truly failures in life. We have found that in most cases, overeating is the only mechanism such a person has for letting go and letting loose the tight reins of control in his or her life. A good example is Larry, a wealthy business-man who is the chief executive officer of a large business. He dresses impeccably, keeps his car perfectly washed and waxed, and lives in a beautifully decorated house in an affluent neighborhood. He maintains rigid discipline with his children and has high expectations for his wife as well. He never drinks or uses drugs; he keeps perfect records of his household finances; and he has an immaculate ap-pointment book that maintains his punctuality. Larry's only outlet from his self-imposed militaristic control is overeating—it is his way of letting off some steam.

Through the Intuitive Eating process, Larry learned to separate his biological hunger from his emotional need for food as a stress reliever. Larry ultimately found other ways to allow himself to let go, such as playing ball with his kids and going disco dancing with his wife. As a result, Larry's compulsive eating lessened and finally all but faded out.

COPING WITH EMOTIONAL EATING

Whether your response to emotional hunger is mild emotional eating or out-of-control bingeing, there are four key steps to making food less important in your life. Ask yourself:

1. *Am I biologically hungry?* If the answer is yes, your next step is to *honor your hunger* and eat! If you are not hungry, answer the following questions.

2. *What am I feeling?* When you find yourself reaching for food when there is no biological hunger, take a time-out to find out what you are feeling. This is not such an easy question to answer, especially if you are not in touch with your feelings. Try the following:

- Write out your feelings.
- Call a friend and talk about your feelings.
- Talk about your feelings into a tape recorder.

- Just sit with your feelings and experience them if you can.
- Talk to a counselor or a psychotherapist.

3. *What do I need?* Many people eat to fulfill some unmet need, which is related to the emotional or physical feeling being experienced. If you are a chronic dieter you can be particularly vulnerable. Eating to assuage an unmet need can be used as an excuse to eat. Here is a simple example:

Molly is a freelance writer who was working into the wee hours to meet her deadline. Around 3:00 in the morning she found herself walking downstairs into the kitchen. She realized that she was not hungry, yet she was about to devour a bowl of ice cream. When Molly asked herself what she was feeling, she discovered frustration, exhaustion, and a sense of being brain-dead. She realized that she was trying to feed both her fatigue and her frustration. But what she really *needed* was rest—no amount of food would replace sleep. She decided to call it a night and go to bed. But before Molly made that decision, she told herself she could have the ice cream tomorrow if she still wanted it. She also realized the ice cream would taste better if she experienced it fully awake rather than half asleep. The next day Molly finished her story and had no desire for the ice cream—she had removed the need.

4. *Would you please . . . ?* It's not unusual to find—when you ask the question "What do I need?"—that the answer can be obtained simply by speaking up and asking for help. Laurel Mellin, innovator of the successful Shapedown weight management program for families, has found that overweight kids often have trouble speaking up for their needs. We find this to be true also for many of our clients. The "Would you please" step originated from Laurel Mellin's work, and we find it extremely helpful for our clients.

Danielle, a full-time stay-at-home mom, learned that she was using food as a momentary time-out. Eating was her only retreat between baby cries. Danielle discovered that what she needed was not food, but time just for herself. To obtain this she used the "Would you please" step. She asked her husband to give her thirty minutes of uninterrupted quiet time after he came home from work. Having gained this, food was no longer so important.

MEETING YOUR NEEDS WITHOUT FOOD

There are various ways in which we learn to handle the unending emotions that life can trigger. Some people learn early on that it's okay to express their feelings or to ask for a hug. Others aren't lucky enough to be taught how to take care of themselves in productive, nurturing ways. The first task in learning how to cope without using food is to acknowledge that you are entitled to having your needs met. But basic needs are often discounted, including:

- Getting rest
- Getting sensual pleasure
- Expressing feelings
- Being heard, understood, and accepted
- Being intellectually and creatively stimulated
- Receiving comfort and warmth

Seek Nurture

Feeling nurtured can allow you to feel comfort and warmth so that food loses its number-one position in this role. There are many routes and avenues available for nurturing yourself and receiving nurturing from others.

- Rest and relax.
- Take a sauna or a jacuzzi.
- Listen to soothing music.
- Take time to breathe deeply.
- Learn to meditate.
- Play cards with friends.
- Take a bubble bath in candlelight.
- Take a yoga class.
- Get a massage.
- Play with your dog or cat.
- Develop a network of friends.
- Ask friends for hugs.
- Buy yourself little presents.
- Put fresh flowers in your house.
- Spend time gardening.

- Get a manicure, pedicure, facial, haircut, etc.
- Get a teddy bear and hug it.

Deal with Your Feelings

If you receive a steady flow of comfort and nurturing you'll be better prepared to face the feelings that have been so frightening. Acknowledge what is troubling you—allow your feelings to come up. This will reduce your need to push them down with food. Here are some suggestions of how to deal with your feelings.

- Write your feelings in a journal.
- Call a friend (or several).
- Talk about your feelings into a tape recorder.
- Release anger through pounding a pillow or a punching bag.
- Confront the person who is triggering your feelings.
- Let yourself cry.
- Breathe deeply.
- Sit with your feelings and discover how the intensity will diminish with time.
- If you have trouble identifying your feelings or coping with them, it may be helpful to talk with a therapist, especially if it is a persistent issue.

Find a Different Distractor

Many people use food as their primary distraction from their feelings. It's okay to get away from your feelings from time to time, *but you don't have to use food as an excuse.* Many teenagers tell us that they come home from school every afternoon and plop down in front of the TV with a bag of chips and a soda. When asked why they do this, they say that they're avoiding the boring feelings of having to do their homework. When it's suggested that they first have a snack to take care of their biological hunger and *then* watch some TV to distract themselves for a while before settling down to homework, they exclaim that their parents would never let them. *As long as they're eating, they can legitimately put off doing home-work, but having other distractors is not allowed!* This is also true for many workaholic clients. It's socially acceptable to take a time-out to eat (a coffee break), but to just sit at the desk, even while entitled to a break, is not allowed. They fear that it will appear as if they are doing nothing. Others use food to distract themselves from loneliness, fear, and anxiety. Since it would be overwhelming to try to feel your feelings twenty-four hours a day, give yourself permission to take a break from them for a while.

Take the assertive stance of distracting yourself in an emotionally healthy way. Try the following:

- Read an absorbing book.
- Rent a movie.
- Talk on the telephone.
- Go to the movies.
- Take a drive.
- Clean out your closet.
- Put on some music and dance.
- Peruse a magazine.
- Take a stroll around the block.
- Work in the garden.
- Listen to a novel on tape.
- Do a crossword puzzle.
- Work on a jigsaw puzzle.
- Play with the computer.
- Take a nap.

HOW EMOTIONAL OVEREATING HAS HURT *AND* HELPED

As you begin to examine your use of food as a coping mechanism, it's helpful to take a look at how food has actually helped you. The notion that overeating can have benefits may sound crazy to you, especially if you're feeling distressed by this behavior and by your weight. *But if there were no up side to overeating, you probably wouldn't continue it.* Take a piece of paper and divide it in half. On one half, make a list of "How using food serves me"—cite all the benefits you receive from overeating. Title the other side, "How using food does me a disservice," and examine the ways in which food has become harmful or destructive to you. A list might look like the following:

How Using Food Serves Me:	How Using Food Does Me a Disservice:
•It tastes good.	•It makes me overweight.
•It's reliable—it's always there.	•My clothes don't fit.
•It keeps me from feeling bored.	•I'm uncomfortable walking and exercising.
•It soothes me.	•My cholesterol is high.
•It numbs my bad feelings.	•I'm numbed to the joys of life.

As you look over your list, you might be surprised to learn that the use of food is not just a negative experience for you. In fact, it may give you some valuable perks. But if you're feeling bad and guilty about using food to cope, it will be hard for you to recognize that its benefits may equalize its burdens. By recognizing that there are indeed some benefits to using food, you'll begin to own your eating experience rather than feeling out of control.

WHEN FOOD IS NO LONGER IMPORTANT

Many clients have talked about having strange, uncomfortable feelings when they're no longer using food to cope with their emotions. At the same time, they're feeling happy and secure in their new Intuitive Eating style and may be losing the weight that has always been a struggle for them. There are a couple of reasons for the conflicting feelings.

• You no longer have the "benefits" of using food. While coping with food can be destructive, one client noted that on tough days she knew she could always go home to her chocolate. Now, instead, she's "stuck" with experiencing her feelings. You might even need to go through a grieving period for the loss of food as comforter and companion.

• You may also notice that you're experiencing your feelings in a deeper, stronger way. Since you're no longer covering them up with food, they may have a profound effect on you. This is a point at which some people decide that it would be helpful to get counseling as a way to process these long-buried feelings.

Sandy is a client who experienced the loss of using food as a coping mechanism. By acknowledging what food used to do *for* her as well as *against* her, Sandy was able to understand that her uncomfortable feelings were normal and appropriate. Sandy had either dieted or used food to cope all of her life. She talked about feeling very frustrated when she would stop eating after finding the threshold bite and truly not wanting any more food. She knew that she'd had enough, didn't want to feel uncomfortable by eating more, yet felt unhappy that she wouldn't be able to continue to have the taste sensations that the food provided. She also talked about feeling angry that she no longer had food to turn to when she was feeling bad. Eating isn't as exciting as it used to be when Sandy would restrict and then overeat. Soon, however, after mourning the loss of being able to *use* food, she was able to leave these feelings behind and feel mainly the exhilaration of being an Intuitive Eater who copes without using food.

A STRANGE GIFT

You may go for a long time without using food to cope, when all of a sudden emotional eating catches you by surprise. If this occurs, it's not a sign of failure or that you've lost ground; instead, it's a strange gift. Overeating is simply a sign that stresses in your life at that moment surpass the coping mechanisms which you have developed. Some of these stresses are divorce, a job change, a move to a new city, the death of someone close, marriage, or the birth of a child. These may be new or unexpected experiences for you. As a result, you haven't had the opportunity to develop coping skills to deal with them. So, you revert to eating as the familiar way to take care of yourself.

Overeating can also recur when your lifestyle becomes unbalanced with too many responsibilities and obligations, with too little time for pleasure and relaxation. Consequently, food is used to indulge, escape, and relax (albeit briefly). When you find this happening, it may be a signal for you to reevaluate your life and find ways to put more balance into it. If you don't make these necessary changes, food remains important by filling an unmet need.

In both of these situations we've described, overeating becomes a red flag that lets you know that something isn't right in your life. Once you truly appreciate this, eating will not feel out of control—rather it's an early warning system. Recognize how lucky you are to have this mechanism to alert you that something is out of kilter in your life! (At first, our clients think this notion is a bit absurd, until they realize the truth behind it in their own lives.) Those people who have never had an emotional eating problem often have no recognizable warning of excess stress in their lives. If you can see that your eating problem can have benefits as well as bad effects, you won't slip into a pattern of self-defeating behaviors that become destructive and difficult to reverse.

USING FOOD CONSTRUCTIVELY

Once you learn new ways of coping with your emotions, think about how food can continue to nurture you in a constructive way. You have a right to feel good—and that means not just not feeling stuffed, but also feeling satisfied with your food choices, being healthy now, and reducing future health risks. Your relationship with food will become more positive as you begin to let go of food as a coping mechanism and bring it into your life as a nonthreatening, pleasurable experience. In Chapter 14 we discuss how you can eat healthfully without falling back into the diet mentality. But first you need to learn how to respect your body and appreciate how it feels when you exercise.

Chapter Twelve

PRINCIPLE 8:

Respect Your Body

Accept your genetic blueprint. Just as a person with a shoe size of eight would not expect realistically to squeeze into a size six, it is equally futile (and uncomfortable) to have a similar expectation about body size. Respect your body so you can feel better about who you are. It's hard to reject the diet mentality if you are unrealistic and overly critical of your body shape.

Body vigilance begets body worry, which begets food worry, which fuels the cycle of dieting. So what do you do, just forget it? Crawl into a dark cave, hide from the world and eat everything in sight? No. But as long as you are at war with your body it will be difficult to be at peace with yourself and food. With every disparaging glance in the mirror, the Food Police gain power, and with that comes vows of just one more diet.

Has all the self-loathing because of your body helped? Has dwelling on your imperfect body parts helped you to become leaner, or merely made you feel worse? Does chewing yourself out every time you step on the scale make your weight any less? We have yet to find one client who says that focusing on his or her body in such negative ways is helpful. Studies have shown that the more you focus on your body, the worse you feel about yourself. Yet the body torture game goes on—Mirror, mirror on the wall, who's the slimmest of them all?

It's hard to escape the body torture game when the whole country is playing it. In the name of fitness, a lean and hard shape has become the body icon for the nineties. Self-proclaimed fitness gurus insist that you can "sculpt" your body as if it were a lump of clay, that you can change your genetic shape with an aerobic huff and puff. We are ardent advocates of being fit and recognize the health benefits of exercise, but we feel we must point out that unrealistic expectations are being painted. It is widely accepted in the research community that you cannot spot-reduce (lose fat in just one specified place). So how could it be that you can sculpt your body by working on certain body parts? Yes, you can build specific muscles through strength and resistance training. And yes, you can lose overall body fat through aerobic exercise. But you cannot personally select where that fat will be lost. It's possible to build muscle underneath fat layers, but this is not the concept of body sculpting that most over-weight people have in mind. Most clients we speak with take body-sculpting classes in hopes of chiseling off the fat.

The fashion world has shaped the ideal look for women into various versions of thin—from the sixties Twiggy figure to the mod-ern waif look embodied by supermodel Kate Moss. Even the full-bodied fashion look turns out to be too thin by medical standards. When clothing giant Guess hired model Anna Nicole Smith, she made headlines in the fashion and news media because she was "big." She weighed 150–155 pounds (gasp), yet was 5' 11", which is in the lower range of ideal according to 1990 U.S. height and weight charts! If a normal weight is considered "big," what does that say about the average woman? This hardly fosters realistic body-shape expectations.

If the ideal body type for women is sandwiched between the Spandex fitness look and fashionable waifness, most bodies don't stand a chance. No wonder body dissatisfaction has become the norm in this country. Repeatedly we seem to be sold the message, If they can do it, you can do it; just try harder (after all, even if you are lean, you could still be leaner). With such standards, it's no wonder that women—and increasingly men, too—are at war with their bodies. Whether you are male or female, fat is the enemy.

There is no doubt that there are unrealistic pressures to be thin, with contributions from the media, advertisers, fashion industry, beauty industry, and on and on. And there are a myriad of cultural factors that lead to unrealistic body expectations. We could groan and point fingers at the causes leading to increased body dissatisfaction. But we want to get past the cause and effect analysis, and instead focus our energy on how to get past body vigilance. Besides, plenty of good books have been written on this topic.

BODY IMAGE: A WAIST IS A
TERRIBLE THING TO MIND

Most of our clients are adept at being overly critical or hating their bodies. And putting an end to body worry and self-loathing is no easy task. Most of us have trouble accepting a compliment, let alone the idea of accepting our bodies. We have found that the notion of accepting your body was too much of a stretch for our clients as a beginning point. They feared that if they accepted their current body size, it would mean complacency, giving up, and getting even bigger. It's one thing to lose the battle of the bulge, they'd say, but to totally give up would mean ultimate failure. At least there's honor and dignity in continuing the fight. Our clients also argued that embracing the notion of body acceptance felt hypocritical. After all, the reason they sought our help is because they did *not* accept their current body—they wanted a change.

What a paradox. Our experience has shown us that to eventually get to your *natural* ideal weight, you need to loosen up on yourself and treat your body with respect.

Remember, repeated diets and a disparaging attitude toward your body have not helped—it's part of what got you to where you are right now. When you are caught in the I-hate-my-body mind-set, it's all too easy to keep delaying good things for yourself, waiting until you have a body that is more deserving. But that day never comes (especially when your standards are unreachable). So you put off treating yourself better. Many aspects of your life literally get weighted down. "I'll join the health club after I lose ten pounds," "I'll go on a special vacation after I reach my goal weight," "I'll start going out with my friends when I just get some of this weight off " — and so the empty promises go. And life gets a little emptier during these times.

Body image expert and psychologist Judith Rodin notes in her book *Body Traps,* *"You don't need to lose weight first in order to*

*take care of yourself. In fact, the process actually happens quite in
the reverse!"* We also have found that if you are willing to make
weight loss a secondary goal and respecting your body a primary
goal, it will help move you forward.

*We are not saying disregard your body—we are urging you
instead to respect it.* This does not mean that you should throw in
the towel. This does not mean that you should disregard your health.
In fact, respecting your body *means* taking care of your health. It is
the beginning, however, of making peace with your body and your
genetics. It is probably the most difficult thing that you will do. If
you can place your priorities on making peace with your food and
body (becoming an Intuitive Eater), it will allow you to loosen up.
Otherwise, it will be a constant tug of war.

It's normal to feel panicky when thinking about respecting your
body. But by doing so it will allow you to go through the Intuitive
Eating steps much more easily. Ironically, we observe a marked
difference between our clients who are able to respect their bodies
and those who are not. Those who are able to get to a place of
respect for their bodies have more patience for the Intuitive Eating
process. This patience allows them to explore further, and move
forward quicker.

Those who have trouble respecting their bodies often find themselves in conflict. When they feel loathsome toward their bodies
they struggle with an intense desire to diet and "just get the weight
off." Then they vacillate with intermittent feelings of peace when
working through the Intuitive Eating process. It is those moments
of peace that give them hope, however, to continue Intuitive Eating.

WHY "RESPECT"

We chose the word *respect* carefully as a launching point for working
through your body issues. It's a tough place to begin for most of
our clients. Just keep in mind these few points, which will ease you
into the idea of body-respect: You don't have to like every part of
your body to respect it. In fact, you don't have to immediately accept
where your body is now to respect it. *Respecting your body means
treating it with dignity, and meeting its basic needs.* Many of our

clients treat their pets with more respect than their own bodies— they feed them, take them out for walks, and are kind to them. Finally, if you are someone who has used food as a way to cope with your emotions over a lifetime, your present body shape may be representative of the way you took care of yourself when you knew no other way. Rather than demeaning the results of this coping mechanism, respect yourself for surviving.

Respecting your body is a critical turning point in becoming an Intuitive Eater. It's not easy. Our culture has a built-in bias against large body sizes while placing a premium on appearance. It's important to recognize that these biases exist, because it may seem like you are a salmon swimming up against the cultural norm. After all, it's all around us in both subtle and blatant forms, from the thin actresses in diet soft drink ads to glaring magazine covers such as *People Magazine*'s January 1994 issue, "Diet Winners and Sinners of the Year: Here's the skinny on who got fat, who got fit and how they did it." It takes a conscious effort to move away from this societal norm. Just because seeking a slender body is the societal norm, does not make it right.

How to Respect Your Body

Think of respecting your body in two ways: first, by making it comfortable, and second, by meeting its basic needs. You deserve to be comfortable. You deserve to get your basic needs met. Or the more miserable you feel, the more miserable you'll be.

Consider these basic premises of body respect:

- My body deserves to be fed.
- My body deserves to be treated with dignity.
- My body deserves to be dressed comfortably and in the manner I am accustomed to.
- My body deserves to be touched affectionately and with respect.
- My body deserves to move comfortably.

Let's explore how you can offer more respect to your body (and to yourself). It's an easy concept to understand, but far more difficult to implement. The following ideas and tools have helped our clients begin a new relationship with their bodies.

Get Comfortable. Let's get personal here. When is the last time you bought new underwear? Don't laugh. All too often we have clients who feel that they don't deserve new underwear (let alone, new clothes) until they reach a certain weight or clothing size. Think about what that means at a basic level. Wearing panties, a bra, or briefs that are constantly pinching or riding up is highly uncomfortable. How can you be at ease in your body when you have a constant unpleasant reminder of your size? Even an old car still needs a new set of tires. While initially you may snicker at the simplicity of changing your underwear, it's had a significant impact on many of our clients. "I just had a baby a few months ago. My maternity underwear was laughably big, but my regular panties fit too snugly. They were a constant reminder that *I* was too big. I felt miserable, until I invested in underwear that fit. The funny thing is that I didn't want to spend the money—even though I had shelled out plenty on a weight-loss program that did not work. I was amazed at how a simple act made such a difference in feeling better about myself."

Cassandra was in her fifties, and hadn't bought new bras in years. (The ones she had were of very high quality and quite expensive, so they had lasted.) Sadly, the underwires in her bras were jabbing and scarring her, but she didn't feel she deserved to buy new bras until she lost weight. Yet every day she was miserable. Her first step toward respecting her body was to buy new bras and pantyhose. Although she knew it would be a while before she reached her ideal, but realistic, weight, she learned that wearing a tortuously tight undergarment would not make the process happen any quicker. When she was more relaxed in her underwear, she was able to be more relaxed about her eating.

The comfort principle goes beyond undergarments. How you dress can be a step toward a newfound respect for your body. We are not saying you should be a slave to the fashion industry, however. Rather, dress in the manner in which you are accustomed. If you are used to dressing in a tailored suit ensemble, why should you stop just because your body is not where you currently want it to be? You should not have to settle for leftovers or dowdy duds. There's nothing wrong with dressing in worn-out jeans and an oversized shirt *if that is what you are used to and comfortable in.* If, however, you prefer wearing dress pants and a casual blazer and settle for worn-out jeans instead, it may affect how you feel about yourself and your body. It's an issue of being consistent. All too often weight-loss programs urged you to "get rid of your fat clothes"; otherwise, they warn, you are issuing an invitation for failure. By following this dictum, however, you are setting yourself up to feel uncomfortable and more body-phobic. Instead, dress for your here-and-now body; be comfortable.

Change Your Body-Assessment Tools. We have found that most of our clients who weigh themselves frequently have difficulty living in their present body—they get too worried about the numbers. Our advice: Stop weighing yourself. Remember, the scale is the tool of a chronic dieter.

Also, beware of substituting a tight pair of jeans as a pseudo-scale or body assessment tool. Hanging on to a small piece of clothing and trying it on daily or weekly can equally undermine how you feel about yourself and your body. Jamie, a young account executive for a public relations firm, was doing quite well with Intuitive Eating. She quit dieting, honored her hunger, respected her fullness, and so forth. Jamie had also gotten rid of the scale. But she began to assess her progress by trying on a tight mini skirt. Every time she tried the skirt on she felt bad about herself. It conveyed the message "You haven't made enough progress. You are still too fat." Jamie eventually got rid of the skirt and her bad feelings about her body. *Even a slender person will feel fat in a pair of pants that feel too tight.*

Quit the Body-Check Game. Most of our clients are embarrassed to admit this, but when they enter a room with other people, they play the silent game of body-checking. The game of body-checking revolves around the theme, How does my body compare to the rest of the crowd? Perhaps you've played this game (and maybe are not even quite aware of it): Am I the fattest one here? Who's got the best body? How does my body rate compared to the others? This can be a dangerous game, especially when played with people you don't know.

We've had clients admire and envy a stranger's body shape. "Oh, if I only had *her* body. She must work out daily. Look at her eat—

only low-fat food. I should be able to do that. Something is wrong with me. I need to try harder." These are big assumptions. You do not know how someone acquired her current body shape. You may not be on a level playing field. You don't know if the person is truly eating! The person may have had surgery (such as liposuction), may suffer from an eating disorder, may have just finished a quickie diet with fast results, and so on. You can't judge the shape of someone's body and assume he or she "earned" it. The person may put on a "false food face" socially. The individual you are admiring may also be miserable in her body! Or this person could just be naturally lean—with no effort at all.

In one session, Kate described a party she had attended and how good a particular woman's body looked. Kate thought that she should be able to get those kind of results too, if she just tried harder. Little did Kate know, however, that the acquaintance at the party was a client of mine (ET), who happened to be bulimic! (Of course, Kate would never know this from me because of strict patient confidentiality.) Kate had been admiring a woman with an eating disorder who was fighting for recovery. The bottom line is, you never know. Even if it is a friend or relative, you still don't know. We have worked with clients whose own spouses and roommates did not know that they had an eating disorder.

Playing the body-check game may lead to more dieting and more body dissatisfaction, as illustrated in the Case of the Dueling Dieters:

Both Sheila and Cassie had been on their share of diets, and they silently competed in the body-check game. This began to change when Sheila became an Intuitive Eater. Sheila had made substantial progress over six months, but her weight was moving much slower than she desired. Fortunately, Sheila accepted this process and was feeling good. Meanwhile, her neighbor, Cassie, had just finished another crash diet. Cassie was proud of her weight loss and paraded her body around. Sheila was beginning to wish her body had changed just as quickly.

That night, Sheila and Cassie went out together for dinner with their husbands. Sheila ate what she wanted, had a good meal, left some food on her plate and over all, felt satisfied. Meanwhile, Cassie proudly nibbled like a bird, while she preened and boasted how easy her current diet was. Next to Cassie, Sheila felt like she was overeating. But she kept listening to her Intuitive Eater voice that told her to respect her body, that her body deserved to be fed, that she should be patient. Her voice gently reminded her that Cassie was on a path to diet destruction—the weight-loss euphoria wouldn't last long. Sheila knew this all too well from her old dieting days.

Sheila's private body competition with Cassie made her feel inferior about her own body and progress. Nonetheless, she continued the journey of Intuitive Eating. One month later, Cassie had gained back all her weight and was binge-eating in spurts. One year later, Sheila was at her natural ideal weight and Cassie was on another diet. But Sheila had come very close to going back on a diet because of playing the body-check game.

Don't Compromise for the "Big Event." Whether it's a class reunion, or wedding, it's natural to want to look your best at important occasions. It's a subtle form of body-checking. But if you succumb to the pressure by "dieting down" to squeeze into that special outfit, it will only backfire. You'll only add another notch on the belt of yo-yo dieting, even if this time it's yo-yo dieting with a cause.

Remember, there will always be important occasions in your life. One particular client was attending the Grammy Awards because her husband was up for an award. Of course she wanted to look not just good, but great. It became clear, however, that she would not be at her ideal body weight for this prestigious event. She was feeling desperate and considered a quick fast to get her weight down. She was asked when will the dieting stop. There will always be an important award or event, always a "legitimate" reason to diet. At that moment she saw the future futility of crash diets triggered by competitive body-checking. She decided to respect her current body. She kept her usual standards of dress and wore a custom-made outfit. This time, however, the outfit was designed for her here-and-now body. She did not have to squeeze into a gown and worry about every move she made. She still maintained her other routine standards—stylish hair-do, glittery accessories, and so forth. The only thing different was that this time she felt comfortable rather than self-conscious.

It's all too easy to cross over into the dieting mentality if you rationalize that the specialness of an event makes it okay to diet. The more you exert pressure on yourself to be a certain body size, the more you are bound to create problems. Jesse would always panic when a special occasion arose, whether it was a wedding or her company's annual awards banquet when she had to give a keynote speech. First, she would worry about what to wear, which would lead her on an intense shopping foray. Eventually, she would buy a stunning dress that was just a little too small. Jesse always shopped for her "future body," rather than her here-and-now body. But she knew she could "make weight" for the big day, just like a boxer weighing in for the big fight. As the big day drew near, Jesse would feel more pressure. She'd try her dress on daily and chastise herself for not fitting into it. Then the meal skipping would begin. On the big day itself, Jesse would allow herself a light breakfast. She would forgo eating the rest of the day to make sure she looked good and fit into her dress. Yes, the dress would fit. But by the time Jesse reached her destination she would invariably overeat (discreetly, of course) at the special function. Her body was famished, and she'd rationalize that she had earned it. But by the end of the night, her overfull stomach would "remind" her she was too big. She'd spend the event worrying about her body rather than having a good time.

How much time and energy have you spent getting your body ready for the big event? What if the energy was directed on recognizing your inner qualities, such as wit, intelligence, or listening ability? What if you came prepared for a function by spending your time thinking of ways to engage in meaningful conversation, or getting to know someone new? You'd probably have a better time! Gladys almost skipped her twenty-year class reunion because she was too big and had nothing to wear. She could not bear the thought of shopping for a larger dress size. Eventually, Gladys decided to put her body worries aside and attend her reunion. Instead of worrying about her body, Gladys focused on finding out what her chums had been doing over the years. She even danced the night away with old friends. (She had not danced in years!) Gladys's reunion experience far exceeded her expectations. She found her "old self"—the witty and charming person that loved to have fun and dance. Over the years, Gladys's private body-war had only served to isolate her and keep her from doing the activities she enjoyed. The sad irony is that Gladys came so close to avoiding her reunion because her body was not ready for the big event. It might have taken Gladys a lot longer to rediscover her wonderful self.

Stop Body-Bashing. Every time you focus on your imperfect body parts it creates more self-consciousness and body worry. It's difficult to respect your body when you are constantly chastising yourself for looking the wrong way. How often do you have these kinds of thoughts?

- I hate my thighs.
- My arms are too fat and wobbly.
- My butt is disgusting.
- I hate my double chin.
- My stomach is gross.

Many of our clients are surprised at how often they degrade their bodies in one day. How many times a day do you chide yourself about your body? Try keeping count for a day or a few hours. It is surprising how often we can be triggered to worry about our body, whether it's a quick glimpse in a store window reflection or passing a mirror. Each disparaging thought lands another nail in the coffin of body dissatisfaction. Surrounding yourself with these body thoughts, will only make you more unhappy and frustrated. It can also bleed over into how you feel about yourself in general.

Instead of focusing on what you don't like about your body, find parts of your body that you do like or at least tolerate. Start simple. Perhaps you like your eyes or smile. We've had clients who could find only one body part they did not dislike, such as their wrist or ankle. That's okay; it's a beginning. Every time you catch a maligning body thought, disarm it. Replace it with a kind body statement that you believe, such as, "I like my smile."

Instead of:	Replace with This Positive Statement:
My puffy jowls are disgusting.	I like my hair.
My thighs are too big.	I like my muscular calves.

If you find saying that you "like" some part of your body is too difficult, try respectful statements.

Instead of:	Replace with This Respectful Statement:
I can't stand my cellulite-dimpled legs.	I'm lucky I have legs that can move my body.
My body is so out of shape, it's horrible.	My body got me to school. I've been supporting my family while finishing my degree, so it was hard to workout optimally.

Respect Body Diversity, Especially Yours. It's ironic that we are celebrating cultural diversity, but as a culture we still have trouble with the idea of body diversity. We come in all shapes and sizes, yet we somehow expect that we should all be one size fits all, as long as it's thin. As long as we feed into this cultural stigma, it will be a long time before societal norms will change into a healthy acceptance of body diversity.

There are many factors that can cause obesity, including genetics, activity level, and nutrition. You cannot assume, for example, that just because someone is overweight he or she earned every ounce with a spoon in one hand and a fork in the other. Several studies have documented that obese people do not necessarily eat more than their lean counterparts. Yes, there are compulsive eaters. Yes, there are those who are not active. But we cannot assume that someone with a large body overeats and does not move. Many classic studies on twins have shown that genetics plays a powerful role in determining our body build.

Obesity is the last bastion where overt prejudice exists. Some call it weightism, others call it fattism, but by any name there is prejudice against people with bigger body sizes. Today it would be unconscionable to make a racial slur, yet body-size slurs abound. When you see a big person on the street, do you cast judgment and disdain? If you are that harsh on a stranger, how can you create a kinder environment for yourself? If you have trouble being kind and respectful to your body, perhaps you can begin with others.

Beware of stereotyping overweight people. Remember that fat people are not any less intelligent, less capable, less well-adjusted, or more gluttonous than thin people. Try beginning with a place of neutrality and compassion. Check your body bias at the door.

While we have spent a great deal of time (and many words) on respecting bigger body sizes, it's important to recognize that some people are naturally born with a leaner body type, although they are in the minority. Similarly, we cannot assume that because someone is fashionably slender he or she has an eating disorder or is obsessed with dieting.

Be Realistic. If maintaining or obtaining your weight requires living on rice cakes and water while exercising for hours, that's a glaring clue that your goal is not realistic. If your parents are extremely heavy, chances are you will never be model-thin. Remember, genetics is a strong determinant of body size.

Do Nice Things for Your Body. Your body deserves to be pampered and touched. Schedule massages as often as you can, even if it's just a fifteen-minute neck rub. Try a sauna or a whirlpool. Buy luxurious smelling lotions and creams to rub on your body. Take bubble baths with bath oils and salts. (Try this in candlelight with classical music!) Doing these things for your body shows that you respect it and want to make yourself feel good.

REACHING YOUR NATURAL
HEALTHY WEIGHT

One of the first questions we are invariably asked is, Can you help me lose weight? Or, How much should I weigh? That answer varies from individual to individual, and is clear only after we've asked several questions. No one can really say what a specific ideal weight is. In fact, the makers of the 1990 U.S. Dietary Goals got rid of an important word when recommending body weights for Americans: *ideal*. They threw out the recommendation that Americans reach or maintain an *ideal weight* because no one knows exactly what that number is! In their updated weight tables, they provide for a broad range of suggested weights according to your height and age (see table on page 178). While these numbers help to set your weight at a healthy level, the ranges can span forty pounds. That's why in part we use the concept of *natural healthy weight*. This is the weight your body will maintain with *normal* eating and *normal* exercise. It's a personalized ballpark weight goal, which considers your weight and dieting history.

The problem with most of the people we see is that their relationship with food is *not normal* due to years of dieting. If you fluctuate between periods of dieting and overeating, you can probably reach your natural healthy weight. If you've been using food to cope with life's ups and downs, you can probably reach your natural healthy weight. *But your healthy natural weight may not match what you have in mind*. The weight that many people wish to achieve or maintain often has more to do with aesthetics than health. According to the National Institutes of Health, many people in this country who do not need to lose weight are trying to—and it may be in part from chasing an unrealistic body size.

A 1992 study demonstrated that a woman's ideal body image is 13 to 19 percent *below* expected weight (which is calculated by dividing actual weight against weight charts determined by the Society of Actuaries tables). This conclusion was drawn by examining the weights of Miss America contestants and *Playboy* centerfolds. Over the years from 1959 to 1988, their weights and body sizes got *thinner*. That level of thinness overlaps with one of the criteria for anorexia nervosa—body weight below 15 percent of expected. If the cultural ideal for women overlaps with eating disorder criteria, American women are not only chasing an unrealistic body goal, but are engaged in a potentially dangerous pursuit.

It's time to get realistic with your weight expectations. To help you do that, begin by answering the following questions (that apply):

SUGGESTED WEIGHTS FOR ADULTS

Height[1]	Weight in pounds[2,3]	
	19 to 34 years	35 years and over
5'0"	[3]97–128	108–138
5'1"	101–132	111–143
5'2"	104–137	115–148
5'3"	107–141	119–152
5'4"	111–146	122–157
5'5"	114–150	126–162
5'6"	118–155	130–167
5'7"	121–160	134–172
5'8"	125–164	138–178
5'9"	129–169	142–183
5'10"	132–174	146–188
5'11"	136–179	151–194
6'0"	140–184	155–199
6'1"	144–189	159–205
6'2"	148–195	164–210
6'3"	152–200	168–216
6'4"	156–205	173–222
6'5"	160–211	177–228
6'6"	164–216	182–234

[1]Without shoes.
[2] Without clothes.
[3] The higher weights in the ranges generally apply to men, who tend to have more muscle and bone; the lower weights more often apply to women, who have less muscle and bone.

USDHH. Dietary Guidelines for Americans, 3rd ed. Home and Garden Bulletin No. 232, 1990.

1. What was your weight:
   In high school _____
   In college _____

2. What's your lowest *stable* weight *without* dieting? _____

3. How does your body build compare to your parents'? _____

4. Dieting weight:
What's the lowest weight you've attained? _____
For how long? _____
What did it take to achieve this weight, any drastic measures? _____
After initial weight loss, what body weight do you return to? _____

5. What's your highest weight? _____

Look at the numbers, except for dieting and highest weights. How do they compare with your current goal? If the numbers are similar, you are in the realm of a realistic goal. If your goal allows for a range, rather than one single magic number, that too is more realistic. If, however, your numbers are vastly different, there's a good chance that you are striving for a goal that's not achievable without harming your body (or mind). Remember, new research shows that the actual process of dieting, losing or recycling the same fifteen pounds, is probably more harmful than the actual body weight itself.

The dieting weight number sheds information on how low your body weight can go under duress, which is *not* realistic. The more extreme the method used to lose weight, such as fasting, the less likely it is that you can rely on that weight as a goal.

You can see how we use this information by looking at Blanche's weight history. Blanche has been dieting since age five, and in adulthood her highest weight was 250 pounds. Blanche's lowest stable weight as an adult was 160. Both her parents are large. Even on stringent medical fasts, Blanche would only weigh 140 for a brief moment, until she resumed eating real food. Although Blanche felt big in high school at 160 pounds, she recognizes that today 160 would not only be a healthy weight to aim for, she'd be thrilled with it.

SAYING GOOD-BYE TO THE FANTASY

One of the hardest facts many of our clients face is that their weight expectations are not realistic for their bodies. Our clients do not like to hear this. For some, it shatters a lifelong dream. But we refuse to perpetuate an unobtainable goal. We will not be partners in helping someone destroy his or her metabolism or health. It would be like giving a cigarette to a smoker.

For example, Kathy is a thirty-year-old actress who came in because she was told to lose weight by her agent. She reported healthy eating habits, with no use of food emotionally, and said she worked out daily for one hour. After a soul-searching session, it was concluded that Kathy not only did not need to lose weight, but doing so would be detrimental to her metabolism and psyche. At 5′4″ and 140 pounds, she was within a healthy weight range even though her weight was higher than society's expectations. She was actually relieved to hear this; she decided she would change agents, and keep looking for jobs until someone would cast her as she was—a healthy person.

Many of our clients discover in hindsight that had they *accepted* the initial body weight that was the cause of their first diet, they'd be happy with that very same weight today! Instead, they've dieted their bodies to a bigger size. So often we hear: "If only I knew then what I know now. I thought I was heavy in high school; now I'd kill for *that* body weight."

You may need to mourn for the lost body you never had or will have, and evaluate what this means to you. What price have you paid (energy, time, emotional investment) chasing one diet after another to seek your fantasy body shape? By saying farewell to the fantasy, you open the door to being at peace not only with your body, but with other *facets* of your life.

Chapter Thirteen

PRINCIPLE 9:

Exercise—Feel the Difference

Forget militant exercise. Just get active and *feel* the difference. Shift your focus to how it feels to move your body, rather than the calorie-burning effect of exercise. If you focus on how you feel from working out, such as energized, it can make the difference between rolling out of bed for a brisk morning walk or hitting the snooze alarm. If when you wake up, your only goal is to lose weight, it's usually not a motivating factor in that moment of time.

If you were to classify your attitude toward exercise, would it be "just-do-it" or "just-forget-it"? Many of our clients fall into the latter category. They are burned out. Working out often went hand-in-hand with the negative experiences of ineffective dieting. Our clients were *not* enjoying exercise for two key reasons. Either they had started exercising when they initiated a diet, or they abused their bodies with unrealistic amounts of exercise, which led to injuries. Regardless, they really felt guilty for not doing enough.

If you began an exercise program while simultaneously starting a diet, it's likely that your energy (calorie) intake was too low. When you don't have enough energy, exercise is not invigorating, let alone fun. It becomes a chore, pure drudgery. When you are underfed from dieting, it's increasingly difficult to exercise, especially if carbohydrates are inadequate (which is often the case with our chronic dieters).

Carbohydrates are the preferred fuel of exercise. As you can see in the table on carbohydrate power, running two miles uses 50 to 55 grams of carbohydrates. This is the amount of carbohydrates found in three slices of bread. If you regularly limit carbohydrate foods (such as potatoes, bread, and pasta) and then add exercise, you are burdening the body with a carbohydrate deficit. Remember,

ESSENTIAL CARBOHYDRATE POWER		
Activity	Carbohydrates Burned (grams)	Equivalent (slices of bread)
Running		
2 miles	50–55	3
6 miles	150–170	10–11
26 miles	500–550	33–37
Swimming		
200 meters	12–15	1
1,500 meters	90–100	6
Cycling—1 hour	230–250	15–17

Adapted from D.L. Costill, Carbohydrates for exercise: Dietary demands for optimal performance. *International Journal of Sports Medicine* 9:5 (1988).

for normal biological functions, the body *must* have carbohydrates. If you do not feed your body enough carbohydrates, it will dismantle its muscle protein to create vital energy. This has been demonstrated even in studies on endurance athletes. Endurance athletes who did not get enough carbohydrates for their exercise activity, burned branched chain amino acids (a component of protein) to help create vital energy to fuel their bodies.

Keep in mind that even very fit and motivated athletes have difficulty working out if they are low on carbohydrates! This effect was illustrated in a study of elite college swimmers by exercise physiologist David Costill of Ball State University in Indiana. He found that swimmers who did not eat enough carbohydrates were *not* able to complete their workouts. If top athletes had trouble working out because they didn't eat enough, why would you expect to be any different?

If you have never enjoyed exercise, let alone experienced the "runners high" euphoria from working out, there's a good chance it was because of dieting, or the diet mentality of limiting foods. When a diet fails, exercise often stops because it was only done as an adjunct to dieting. You are left with memories of feeling bad, which makes you less likely to want to exercise in the future.

No wonder the chronic dieter has difficulty with consistent exercise. Who wants to continually subject his body to something that does *not* feel good? Yet clients often blame themselves for not having enough willpower, or not possessing the admirable "just-do-it" mantra of exercise. This is like feeling guilty for not having enough willpower to "will" a car to operate on an empty tank of gas. Yet to reap the many positive results from exercise there needs to be a consistent effort.

Many of our clients have been burned out both mentally and physically from "crash exercising." Like crash diets, crash exercising doesn't last long. This typically occurs when someone is determined to get in shape and lose weight quickly. They start with too much activity in a short time period and end up either very sore, or not enjoying exercise, or both.

Others feel intimidated by not having a lean enough body to go to the gym or work out. It's a one-two intimidation punch. First, because they don't feel thin enough next to all the other hard bodies. Second, because they get a glaring self-conscious reminder from floor-length mirrors plastered on every empty wall.

There are other reasons why chronic dieters don't feel like starting or continuing to exercise:

- Bad experiences growing up, including: being forced to run laps or do calisthenics as a punishment, being teased for being uncoordinated, not getting picked for teams.
- Rebelling against parents, spouses, and others who pushed exercise, like a "good" diet: "You should go run," "You should go to the gym," and so forth.

BREAKING THROUGH EXERCISE BARRIERS

Rather than insisting that our clients immediately embark on an exercise regime, we wait until they are ready. Postponing activity for a few weeks, even a few months, will not make a big difference in a lifelong commitment. So, don't worry if you don't feel like tying on your shoes and running a few laps, especially if you have leaned toward being an exercise abuser. There are several keys for breaking through the barriers that prevent you from exercising.

Focus on How It Feels

We have found that one key to consistent exercise is to focus on how it feels, rather than playing the numbers game of counting calories burned. Instead of just biding your time or gritting your teeth when working out, explore how it makes you feel throughout the day (including during exercise and immediately after). How do you feel regarding:

- Stress level—Are you able to handle stress better? Are you less edgy? Is it easier to take situations in stride, roll with the punches?
- Energy level—Do you feel more alert? A little more spunky?
- General sense of well-being—Do you have an improved outlook on life?
- Sense of empowerment—Do you feel more in control? Do you say "I can do it," and seize the day?
- Sleep—Do you sleep more soundly and wake up more refreshed?

If you are in a period of inactivity, it's especially important to note these feelings. They will serve as your baseline. Compare the difference between when you did and did not exercise. Note how you felt. When you can really feel the difference between exercising consistently and being inactive, the positive feelings can be a motivating factor for continuing. Why would you stop doing something that feels good? Instead, if you exercise with the dieting mind-set, you get used to stopping and starting, just like each new dieting attempt. In fact, it has been shown that 70 percent of those who begin an exercise program quit during the first year. Remember, *exercise is much more than a calorie-eating machine.*

Disassociate Exercise from Weight Loss

Are we saying exercise doesn't affect weight loss? No. It's well accepted that physical activity is the one consistent element associated with long-term weight maintenance. Exercise plays a significant role in metabolism and preserving lean muscle mass. Yet exercise alone accounts for only part of weight loss. So if your only focus is on weight loss, it won't motivate you to exercise for long. It will only serve like a time card being punched by a bored assembly-line employee. And when the pay-off isn't quick enough, it could be discouraging. Using weight loss as the ultimate reason for physical activity could also drive you to exercise abuse. Even then, you still may not be happy with your body.

Focus on Exercise as a Way of Taking Care of Yourself

Whether thin or heavy, young or old, everyone benefits from being active. It makes you feel good and helps prevent health problems later in life. Specific benefits include:

- Increased bone strength
- Increased stress tolerance
- Decreased blood pressure
- Reduced risk of chronic diseases, including heart disease, diabetes, osteoporosis, hypertension, and some cancers
- Increased level of good cholesterol (HDL); decreased total cholesterol level
- Increased heart and lung strength
- Increased metabolism—helps maintain lean body mass and revs up energy production in the cells

Don't Get Caught in Exercise Mind Games

If you've had a diet mentality for a number of years, there's a good chance that versions of it have permeated into do-not-exercise traps. Let's identify and refute them:

The It's-Not-Worth-It Trap. We know many people who wouldn't walk unless they could get in one hour—anything under that "doesn't count." Therefore, a fifteen-minute walk break during lunch doesn't count. Instead, they do nothing. We commonly see clients discount their workout because they didn't reach their prescribed quota. It "didn't count" because they only exercised three times in a week, rather than five. All the more reason to be focused on how exercise feels, rather than doing it by the numbers.

Besides, over the long term, it all counts. Since many of our clients are very numbers-oriented, we use numbers to show them how "it matters":

Activity	Time Spent in I Year
5 minutes of taking the stairs at work twice daily/ five times a week	43 hours
10 minutes of walking your child to school three times a week	26 hours
15 minutes of mowing the lawn one time a week	13 hours

Couch-Potato Denial. The classic image of a couch potato is a person leisurely reclined on the couch with the remote control in one hand and a snack or two in the other. However, it's all too easy to lead what we call a "hectic couch-potato lifestyle" without ever laying your body on a sofa. Your life may be very hectic, but *being busy is not the same as physical activity*. Most of us spend time "running around" in our car! Unless you are Fred Flintstone, there is no fitness element to driving. Any of the following could be a component of couch-potato existence:

- Spending hours *sitting* in transit to work (either car, train, bus, taxi)
- Sitting behind a desk all day (pushing papers and fax and telephone buttons is no different than fiddling with the remote control)
- Working at a computer all day
- Arriving home exhausted, then sitting and reading the mail or paying bills, eating, then going to bed

The key is to find ways to incorporate physical activity into your everyday life. Remember, hectic schedules and mental exertion may keep your mind active, but that is not the same.

The No-Time-to-Spare Trap. Ask most people if exercise is important, and you'll get an overwhelming yes. Yet it often gets shoved aside as other details in life vie for your time and attention. This is especially evident when you consider that less than 10 percent of adults in this country regularly engage in physical activity.

The question we often ask our patients who are in this time-crunch dilemma is, "How can you make exercise a nonnegotiable priority?" This is not intended as a rigid guideline, but rather a new way of thinking about exercise so that it won't slip through the cracks.

If this seems like an impossible task, you may need to reevaluate your standards and priorities. Your life may be chronically over-scheduled. Can you continue living this way? If so, what price are you paying? Are you taking care of yourself? Are you happy? Do you feel good? Ironically, many of our overscheduled clients attribute the fact that they don't work out to laziness, when in reality, they are truly too busy! If time is rare and precious, then you certainly cannot afford to be sick. All the more reason to invest in making time to take care of yourself.

An option you may want to explore is hiring a personal trainer, if you can afford it. "When I make an appointment with somebody, including my trainer, it automatically becomes a priority on my schedule," said one client. Be sure, however, to check out the trainer's credentials. Minimally, a personal trainer should be certified through either the American College of Sports Medicine (ACSM) or the American Council on Exercise (ACE).

The If-I-Don't-Sweat-It-Doesn't-Count Trap. It's easy to believe that the only way to be fit is to engage in activities that make you sweat profusely. But you don't have to invest in sweat equity to reap fitness dividends. A surprising but welcome conclusion reached jointly by the Centers for Disease Control (CDC) and the American College of Sports Medicine (ACSM) in 1993 was that you don't have to perform rigorous workouts to be physically fit. You can gain benefits from simple activities such as gardening, raking the leaves, or walking. These no-sweat activities make a physical difference. After reviewing over forty-three studies, the CDC and ACSM concluded that *simply moving* thirty minutes over the course of most days of the week could reduce the risk of heart disease by half!

All you need to do is accumulate thirty minutes of activity a day, most of the week. The thirty minutes of activity do *not* need to be all at once. (This particular conclusion surprises many people.) For example, the activity could be divided into three ten-minute sessions, or two fifteen-minute sessions, and so forth. Every little bit counts!

GETTING STARTED ON A LIFE-LONG COMMITMENT

Get Active in Daily Living

Kids are naturally active—squirming, running, and jumping. But as we get older our physical activity declines in spite of fast-paced living.

Unlike children, we need to consciously look for ways to increase our routine activity. Begin by asking how you can become more active in your daily living. For example, consider parking your car down the block to build in a ten-minute walk to work. When you factor in the return walk, you've just built twenty minutes of walking into your day. Add a ten-minute walk break during lunch and you've met the minimum level for physical fitness and its health benefits. Do this five times a week and you've walked 130 hours, or about 400 to 500 miles in one year! Remember, ordinary activities do make a difference. (Of course, conventional exercise can also be included, such as running or aerobics.)

Get rid of energy-saving devices and invest in human energy that will help you increase your daily activities.

- Use a hand-push lawn mower rather than a power-operated one.
- Take the stairs rather than the elevator.

Make Exercise Fun

For some people this means exercising with a friend, family member, or trainer. It might be the one time of the day you can talk freely with a friend, uninterrupted. Or perhaps your days are so crazed with demands from other people that a little solitude would add to your exercise enjoyment.

One sure way to take the fun out of exercise is to get injured. Do be sure to start slowly in whatever activity you choose. Some further suggestions:

- Be sure to choose activities that you enjoy. Consider playing a team sport such as volleyball, basketball, or tennis.
- Do engage in a variety of activities—you need not dedicate your life to just one sport. By diversifying, you'll also decrease your chance of injuries and increase your enjoyment factor.
- If you exercise at home on stationary fitness equipment, add fun by getting a VCR and taping your favorite soap opera or television movie or reading a good book or magazine (rather than work-related papers).
- Make your walk more enjoyable with a portable cassette player. Listen to books on tape or your favorite music.

Make Exercise a Nonnegotiable Priority

Ask yourself, "When can I consistently make the time to work out?" Make an appointment with yourself to work out, and honor it as you would any other meeting or appointment.

If you travel a lot:

- Pack your walking shoes. (It's an interesting way to get to know a new city.)
- Pack a jump rope. (It's a lightweight piece of equipment that delivers a cardio-wallop in a short amount of time.)
- Choose hotels that have workout facilities. (They are increasing in number.)
- Take advantage of airport layovers and walk around the airport. (It usually feels good after hours of sitting.)

Be Comfortable

Workout attire need not be fashion show material, but it is important to wear clothes that breathe and allow you to move. This also means dressing for the weather. Heavy sweats can make you uncomfortably hot when you wear them to disguise your body. An oversize light-weight T-shirt and leggings will usually do for women. Or bike shorts with an oversize shirt works well for both men and women.

Don't forget about comfortable shoes as well. Not only will they feel good; they are an investment in injury prevention.

Include Strength Training

Strength training helps rebuild muscle wear and tear from dieting. This is also important because our lean muscle mass declines as we get older. Americans lose an average of about 6.6 pounds of lean muscle mass for each decade of life. Therefore, someone who has been dieting for years is losing her muscle tissue from both aging *and* dieting. Remember, muscle is metabolically active tissue that helps keep your metabolism revved up. In fact, Bill Evans and Irwin Rosenberg, Tufts University researchers and authors of *Biomarkers*, estimate that our metabolic rate decreases 2 percent each year from the age of twenty, and they attribute this downward shift of metabolism to decreasing muscle mass.

Ordinary activity, and even vigorous activity such as running, does not leave you immune to muscle-wasting due to age. A ten-year study following master runners (minimum age of forty) showed that while they maintained their fitness from running, they lost an average of 4.4 pounds of muscle from their untrained areas. Their muscles stayed the same size in their legs but decreased in their arms. There was an exception, however, for three runners who did upper body weights. They were able to *maintain* their fat-free weight in their upper body. Therefore, you don't have to lose your muscle mass.

The American College of Sports Medicine (ACSM) recommends that strength training be an integral part of a fitness program for *all* healthy adults. Specifically, they recommend:

- Strength training at least twice a week
- Doing one set of eight to twelve repetitions of eight to ten exercises for conditioning of each of the major muscle groups

BEYOND PHYSICAL FITNESS

Is there anything wrong with wanting to work out more, to burn body fat? No. Just be careful that you do not fall into the dieting-weight loss trap, where you become a slave to working out and counting calories burned. We have found that increasing exercise can be a good way to channel anxiety while becoming an Intuitive Eater. Intuitive eating can feel foreign and slow in the beginning, especially when the world around you is dieting. Exercise allows you to feel that you are actively doing something about your body. You *feel* benefits.

It's one thing to invest several hours in exercise if you are training for a marathon or because you are an athlete. It's a problem, however, when exercise consumes you, and begins to interfere with your everyday living. Exercising more isn't necessarily better. How do you know if you are reaching the outer limits of exercise? Signs of *exercise abuse* include:

- Inability to stop, even when you are sick or injured
- Feeling guilty if you miss a single day
- Inability to sleep at night—a sign of overtraining
- Paying exercise penance for eating too much, such as running an extra three miles because you ate a piece of pie
- Being afraid that you will suddenly get fat if you stop for a single day

RR—REMEMBER REST

The hardest lesson that I (ET) learned as a competitive marathoner was that rest was every bit as important as training. It's also hard for our clients to recognize this tenet of training. Similarly, if for some reason you are unable to work out on a particular day, it does not mean that you will be suddenly out of shape or gain weight.

Some clients fear that once they stop exercising they will not continue. That's the all-or-nothing thinking commonly seen in dieters. There's an easy way to prove to yourself that no exercise today does not mean no exercise forever. Simply resume exercise when you are able. The more you reinitiate an exercise program after a break from it, the more confidence you will have in your ability to continue exercising, even if it's been a few days. After a while it stops being a big issue or worry. Besides, this time it's different. You are not dieting, therefore it will be much easier to resume training.

Remember, a few days or weeks of no exercise will not make or break your health or weight. After the big 1994 Los Angeles earthquake, Diane, a client, had to stop exercising. But for the first time, Diane knew that although three weeks had passed, it wasn't a big deal. She knew she'd be lacing up her walking shoes again in the near future. Diane missed the stress relief; she missed the freedom from the kids. But she also knew that she had a house to rebuild. After the earth settled, she got back to her routine walking. Her missed exercise did not become a crisis, and neither did her weight.

Sometimes, taking care of yourself means choosing *not* to exercise. For example, if you only got four hours of sleep and exercising means rising at five in the morning, it's probably best to take that day off. Remember, rest is important. Likewise, if you feel a cold coming on, or you're feeling worn-out, take a day off. Listen to your body. Rest will also help keep exercise feeling fresh and fun.

Chapter Fourteen

PRINCIPLE 10:

Honor Your Health—
Gentle Nutrition

Make food choices that honor your health and taste buds while making you feel well. Remember that you don't have to eat a perfect diet to be healthy. You will not suddenly get a nutrient deficiency or gain weight from one snack, one meal, or one day of eating. It's what you eat consistently over time that matters. Progress, not perfection, is what counts.

I keep thinking that someday I'm going to walk in here and you're going to tell me the food party is over." We hear this fear a lot. It's one of the reasons that nutrition is discussed with our patients much later in the Intuitive Eating process, rather than sooner. It's also the reason that *honor your health* is the last principle of Intuitive Eating. You can hardly talk about health and taking care of yourself without discussing nutrition. But our experience has shown us that if a healthy relationship with food is not in place first, it's difficult to pursue a truly healthy diet. If you've been a chronic dieter, the best nutrition guidelines can still be embraced like a diet.

We don't want to give the impression that just because nutrition is reserved for the last chapter it's not important. We certainly value health. Don't worry, though—we are not going to pull the food carpet out from under you.

The role of nutrition in preventing chronic disease has been clearly established by the scientific community. But the emerging importance of nutrition has served to breed a nation of "guilty" eaters—feeling the need to apologize for eating a traditional Thanksgiving meal or a fatty dessert.

WHAT IS HEALTHY EATING?

Our whole country needs a food-attitude adjustment. You don't have to be a chronic dieter to be worried about food. Almost daily there is a new headline or cover story on a nutrition-related topic: from killer biotech tomatoes to research proclaiming that margarine is no better than butter (and may be even worse). At best, the dueling headlines get you confused, and at worst, they contribute to a growing food phobia. With special interest groups massaging the media, the fear is magnified. (The alar-apple scare is probably the best example of this.) Add the food companies that climb onto any nutritional bandwagon that furthers their economic cause, and you have a nation of confused and worried consumers.

The medical nutrition research as it's reported in the media easily creates the impression that food will either kill or heal you. This fuels the fire of magical thinking with food. No wonder some people still erroneously believe that eating vinegar or grapefruit will burn off fat. Or that a special food combination is going to raise their metabolism. Sadly, this isn't so.

Ironically, nutrition stories that blow the whistle on misleading food products unintentionally create more fear of food. The message to the consumer is that you can't trust the food companies or the food label—you've been duped. Before the Nutrition Labeling Education Act (NLEA) was implemented, consumers learned that:

- "No-cholesterol" food products such as nondairy creamer were often high in fat.
- Lean-sounding meats such as turkey hot dogs were high in fat.
- "Light" foods were anything but.

It's no surprise that frustrated consumers learned to choose foods about which there is no nutritional doubt—fat-free foods. It's easy to inspect fat grams—just look for the zero. No complicated "fat math" formulas are required to double-check if the food company is living up to its healthy image. However, while the NLEA dramatically eliminated the loopholes allowing misleading food labels, food still remains suspect in the eye of the consumer. Food and fat phobia prevail.

If you are worried about what's in your food, how can you begin to enjoy it? If you believe that a magical food or pill is around the corner to solve your weight issues, why would you even look inward for the answers? If you don't trust what's in your food, and have trouble trusting your body's inner signals for eating, how can you begin to eat healthfully without guilt or trepidation?

Eating healthfully should feel good both physically and psychologically. But we've lost sight of that feeling due to the food and fat phobia that's sweeping the country. Michelle Stacey, author of *Consumed: Why Americans Love Hate and Fear Food*, concludes that Americans need to change their eating attitude to what she calls enlightened hedonism, a balance between information and pleasure, an educated hedging of bets. That's just how we approach nutrition and food.

We define healthy eating as eating primarily healthy food *and* having a healthy relationship with food. Up until now we've focused on the relationship part. If you are still struggling in this area, you may want to wait a while before you read or act on the information in this chapter.

THE TENETS OF FOOD WISDOM

No doubt you've heard for years of the nutritional merits of variety, moderation, and balance. There's a reason these nutrition mantras have been chanted for decades: They work!

"Eat a variety of foods" sounds just like "Wear a sensible pair of shoes"—practical but easily ignored advice. However, it's actually one of the best ways to hedge your bets for healthy eating. A new study looking at diet diversity has gotten those sensible shoes tap dancing in the spotlight of health. According to a study reported in the *American Journal of Clinical Nutrition*, people who omitted several food groups had a higher chance of dying! Adults who ate foods from only two or fewer food groups were associated with an excess mortality risk of 50 percent in men and 40 percent in women. But how often do you eat the same meal day after day? When was the last time you tried a new cereal, or changed the kind of bread you eat?

In the world of dieting, it may have seemed easier and safer just to eliminate foods rather than balancing them into your meals. Or perhaps you've been so afraid that you couldn't eat just moderate amounts of some foods that you just shun them altogether. But where has that gotten you? Here's where the nutritional tenets of moderation and balance can help. First of all, moderation does not mean elimination. If you eliminate whole groups of foods it can be harder to get the nutrients your body needs. Moderation is simply eating various amounts of food without going to extremes of either too little or too much.

Secondly, balance is intended to be achieved over a period of time—it does not have to be reached at each and every meal. Your body does not punch a time clock. Most nutrition recommendations are intended to be an *average* over time, not for a single meal or a single day, and with good reason. You will not suddenly get a nutrient deficiency if you did not eat enough in one day. Similarly, you will not make or break your health or your weight from one meal or even one day of eating. It is consistency over time that matters. Our bodies are remarkably adaptable. Here are a few examples:

- If you eat too little iron, the body starts to absorb *more* of it.
- If you take in too much vitamin C, the body begins to excrete more of it.
- If you eat too little in general, the body slows its need for calories.

MAKING PEACE WITH NUTRITION

Eating nutritiously does not have to be about deprivation, although that's what most Americans fear. A 1993 American Dietetic Association survey of American eating habits revealed that 39 percent of adults said that an obstacle to good nutrition is having to give up favorite foods. It's no surprise that a majority of adults (56 percent) surveyed in a 1990 Gallup poll said they didn't find eating pleasurable at times because they worried about fat and cholesterol. If most people feel that eating healthfully means giving something up, whether it's taste or a favorite food, no wonder nutritious eating seems difficult. Fortunately, it is possible to balance taste and pleasure with healthy eating.

The problem is that healthy eating for many people has been clouded with bad food experiences. How often have you heard, for example, "You'll get used to it"—which really means that the food tastes so bad you have to condition yourself to like it! Or how many times were you told as a child, "Eat your vegetables, then you can have dessert"—which really means that vegetables are so difficult to eat that you deserve a reward for choking them down. Or maybe you've experienced:

- Inferior fat-free foods—fat-free replicas of the real thing—from food companies scrambling to capitalize on the fat-free market. Rubbery fat-free mozzarella and cream cheese that resembles a caulking agent hardly foster enthusiasm for healthy eating.
- "Pretend foods."—This is where you pretend that what you are eating is a terrific substitute for what you'd *really like* to be eating. For example, pretending that you are sipping a rich chocolate milkshake when it's actually a few ice cubes whipped with a diet hot chocolate mix in the blender. Or making do with applesauce adorned with graham cracker crumbs instead of apple pie.

In fact, the combination of taste atrocities in the name of healthy eating with the epidemic fear of food prompted noted chef and cookbook writer Julia Child to take action. In 1990, she spearheaded a revolutionary project through the American Institute of Wine & Food (AIWF) called Resetting the American Table: Creating a New Alliance of Taste and Health. This venture joined together opinion leaders from the culinary world and the health community. Their task was to find out if it is possible to move Americans toward a healthier diet without their having to give up the pleasures of the table. The consensus was an overwhelming yes. Here's some of what they came up with:

- Their umbrella tenet: In matters of taste, consider nutrition, and in matters of nutrition, consider taste.

- Negative, restrictive approaches to eating do not work.
- People need to be steered toward a healthy diet they can live with, *without guilt*.

They also gave guidelines for five core areas that link taste and health: 1) nutrition; 2) physical activity; 3) food availability, quality, and preparation; 4) food safety; and 5) education.

If a food aficionada can consider nutrition without compromising her gastronomic palate, so can you! We call this approach *gentle nutrition*. Taste is important, but health is still honored—without guilt.

PRACTICING GENTLE NUTRITION

Feed Your Metabolism

Clearly, you need to eat. Remember that to stoke your metabolic fire you need wood, not just kindling. For many of our clients, this means eating more of some foods than they are used to, especially carbohydrates. You may be thinking, Forget eating more, I'll just exercise. But as we explained in Chapter 13, exercise alone will not prevent metabolic damage from undereating, even for athletes. Scientists at the University of British Columbia in Canada studied fourteen competitive female rowers. Half of them were weight-cyclers. During the study, the weight-cyclers lost about ten to eleven pounds during the four weeks leading up to their national championships. Consequently, their metabolic rates plummeted by about 7 percent. They also lost over six pounds of fat-free body mass (primarily muscle). In this particular study, the rowers were fortunate and were able to get back their previous metabolic rate *when they began eating more*. If athletes can lose precious muscle from undereating, why would you be any different? Remember, the more muscle you have, the higher your metabolic rate.

How do you go about feeding your body? It's a scary prospect for most of our clients, who are afraid they will gain weight. To help you overcome this fear, keep reminding yourself that by feeding your body you are feeding your metabolism.

Nutritional Guidelines

We use a modified Food Pyramid approach we call the Nutrition Countdown to help establish some minimum nutritional goals. (The Food Pyramid is the latest healthy eating guideline from the government.) We're hesitant to mention serving sizes, lest it rouse your diet mentality. For the sake of assuring a healthy body and metabolism, we will specify them. But, please, do not misconstrue this as a diet. These are not diet rules but *minimum* guidelines, adapted in part from the *smallest* servings recommended in the Food Pyramid. The reason we stress the smallest numbers is that many of our clients have trouble with how large these numbers seem and tend to want to cut down! You do need to eat at least this amount of food each day to be healthy. We've added the "countdown" part (6–5–4–3–2–1) because it's an easy way to remember the minimum food servings needed for health. Remember, though, we're looking at averages over time. So don't worry if your daily eating does not exactly follow this pattern.

Countdown Number of Servings/Day	What's a Serving? (Minimum Amounts)	Food Group
6	½ cup (cooked) 1 slice (breads)	Grains
5	1 cup raw; ½ cup cooked	Fruits/Vegetables
4	1 ounce	Protein
3 (per *week*)	¾ cup (soups) ½ cup beans	Beans
2	1 cup	Dairy or Calcium-rich
1	½ gallon (8 8-oz. glasses)	Water

Grains. The best kind of food to fuel your body is at the base of the Food Pyramid, the complex carbohydrates, found primarily in grains. Carbohydrates serve as the foundation of healthy eating, yet all too often they have been shunted from a chronic dieter's repertoire for fear of getting fat. As we're fond of telling our clients, carbohydrates are your friend! While this may sound a bit trite, our clients find it comforting, especially when carbohydrate-rich foods have been treated like the enemy for so long.

Chronic dieters are not the only ones falling short in carbohydrates. Most Americans don't meet the recommended six servings. Don't let the idea of six servings scare you. If this seems too big a jump from where you are currently eating, begin slowly and build up.

Do choose whole-grain products when possible, such as whole wheat bread, brown rice, and whole grain crackers. Otherwise, it's all too easy to fall short in meeting your fiber needs. In addition, whole grains provide more vitamins and minerals than their refined counterparts. If you are like the average American, you're only getting half the fiber you need. Fiber plays an important role in digestion by helping keep the food moving down the GI tract. The list of the health benefits of fiber keeps growing. Research has shown that different types of fiber play a significant role in preventing chronic diseases such as cancer, heart disease, and diabetes. Insoluble fiber, found primarily in whole wheat products, plays a big role in preventing some types of cancer, especially colon cancer. Soluble fiber, found in oats and beans, plays a role in lowering blood cholesterol and managing blood sugar levels in diabetics. The health benefits from these different types of fibers underscore the value of eating a varied diet.

Fruits and Vegetables. We merged these two groups together, which is consistent with the recommendations from the National Cancer Institute and their 5-a-Day-for-Better-Health campaign. We need to get at least five servings a day from this group. It's not that you have to get five different fruits or vegetables in your diet each day (that could seem overwhelming). Rather, you need to get the minimum number of *servings*—think volume. Generally, a serving size is one-half cup for cooked vegetables or fruit, or one cup raw. For example, here are foods that are equivalent to five servings:

- 2 oranges and 1½ cups salad
- 1 apple and 2 cups cooked broccoli
- 1 cup fruit salad and 1½ cups cooked carrots

One of the reasons fruits and vegetables are so important to health is that research has consistently shown worldwide that people who eat higher amounts of fruits and vegetables have lower rates of cancer. In almost every study looking at plant food and people (at least 150 studies to date), plant food is associated with lowering the risk of cancer. These foods are loaded with antioxidants and fiber, which offer many other health benefits. Plus, there is a growing body of research that shows fruits and vegetables contain special food factors called phytochemicals that have added health benefits. For example:

Phytochemical	Plant Food	Potential Benefit
Limonene	Citrus fruits	Helps increase enzymes that get rid of cancer-causing agents
Sulforaphanes	Cruciferous vegetables: broccoli, cauliflower, brussels sprouts, and cabbage	Helps amplify the body's own defense against chemicals that can lead to cancer
Allyl sulfides	Leeks, garlic, onion, chives	Increases the production of enzymes that make it easier for the body to excrete cancer-causing compounds
Ellagic acid	Grapes	Scavenges carcinogens and may prevent them from altering the body's DNA

There are hundreds and maybe even thousands of phytochemicals. Research is just beginning to scratch the surface on their health benefits. This is one reason why we can't rely on getting all of our nutrition in a bottle. You can't manufacture compounds that have yet to be identified and put them into a supplement!

One problem we've seen with our chronic dieters is that they've been "veggied-out." For example, nearly every diet regimen prescribes celery and carrot sticks as the safe and approved snack of choice. If that's your case, ask yourself how you can incorporate vegetables (and fruit) in a manner that's *pleasing* and does not smack of a weight-loss diet, such as adding grated carrots to a favorite pasta sauce. Think of ways in which you can eat fruits and vegetables as a built-in component to a meal, such as:

- Vegetable lasagna
- Ratatouille
- Potato cakes spiced with various chopped vegetables
- Stir-fried vegetables on rice
- Stuffed baked squash
- Stuffed peppers
- Stuffed baked potatoes
- Fajitas (they're usually loaded with vitamin-rich peppers)
- Pancakes topped with a fresh fruit medley
- Fruit compote
- Fruit smoothie

One client, Sally, was averse to fruit, though she didn't know why; she just had trouble eating it. But one day she found she was having no difficulties whatsoever. What had changed? Two things. First, she was rid of her diet mentality, and second, she began eating fruit in a "nondiet" manner. All of her past diets had prescribed eating a spartan single fruit for a snack or with a meal, such as a plum, an apple, and so forth. When she tried fruit salads of all sorts, her interest in fruit was renewed.

Frankly, we've never seen anyone get into trouble eating fresh fruits and vegetables (unless that's all they eat). In fact, preliminary research results also show this to be true. John Potter, a physician and researcher out of the University of Minnesota, has been studying a group of people who were told to eat up to eight servings a day of fruits and vegetables. His preliminary data suggests that people eating more fruits and vegetables actually like it and *feel better doing it*.

Protein. This nutrient and the group of foods containing it has been highly overrated in the dieting world. We've had several patients "inform" us that they were on high-protein diets to protect their muscles. But if your body is on limited calories and not getting enough energy, it doesn't matter how much protein you eat, the dietary protein will still be converted to energy. Remember, the body must have energy at any cost—this means at the expense of protein in your diet, and protein from your body (muscle). Also, to build muscle you need both adequate calories and exercise. If all it took was protein to build muscles, we'd have a nation of muscle-bound citizens! Americans, on average, get twice the amount of protein that their bodies need.

Protein is important for building and maintaining blood, muscle, and other tissues. It plays a vital role in immunity. And every enzyme in our body is made of protein. But, too much protein could be a problem for women. High-protein diets cause the body to leach calcium from the bones and excrete it in the urine. This might compound the osteoporosis problem that women in this country face. (One out of every four women will develop this thinning-bone problem by the time she reaches age sixty-five.)

It's easy to get enough protein in your diet. The average adult man and woman need only 63 and 50 grams of protein, respectively. Four ounces of lean meat will provide 28 grams of protein. Plus you get protein from the other food groups. See how quickly they add up:

Group	Protein per Serving (Grams)	Average Total per Day (Daily Servings × Grams)
Grains	2	12
Fruits/Vegetables	1	5
Protein	7	28
Beans	7	3
Dairy	8	16
Water	0	0
		64

Beans. While beans are barely given an honorable mention in the traditional Food Pyramid, we believe their special nutritional qualities should garner them more attention. The California Department of Health also feels this way. That's why in their 1990 report, The California Daily Food Guide, they recommended that Californians eat beans three times a week.

Here are a few noteworthy facts about beans. They are:

- Rich in complex carbohydrates
- A good source of protein
- Higher in fiber than most cereals
- Rich in folic acid and iron, both of which are hard-to-get nutrients for women
- Shown to help lower blood cholesterol
- A source of the phytochemicals, isoflavones, phytosterols, and saponins that may help the body fight off cancer-causing reactions

Most of our clients believe that beans, like breads, are fattening. This is not true. In fact, a bean-based meal such as black beans and rice is often much lower in fat and calories than a "regular" meat-based meal. We don't want to emphasize calories here, but it helps to break through this common misperception. Our clients are often surprised how satisfying a bean-based meal can be.

Here are some easy ways to add beans to your meals:

- Add garbanzo beans (chickpeas) or kidney beans to your salads.
- Try bean soups as a meal or snack.
- Try the instant bean soups-in-a-cup for a convenient snack.
- Include beans in a burrito.
- Puree beans as a dip.

Dairy. The importance of this food group is that it contains calcium, which is essential for bone health. While women may be quite aware of the need for calcium, men often feel they no longer need this mineral. Whether male or female, your requirements for calcium don't suddenly stop once you become an adult. Bones may seem like a static, inactive part of your body, but this couldn't be further from the truth. Your bone skeleton gets replaced every five years.

Bone density decreases with age in all people after the age of thirty-five. If you don't get enough calcium from food, it will be leached from bone. Calcium also plays a vital role in many metabolic processes in the body. High-calcium food traditionally means dairy products such as milk, yogurt, and cheese. But for those of you who choose to be strict vegetarians, there are other calcium-rich foods you can have such as kale or collard greens. If this is a problem, consider a calcium supplement.

Water. Water is essential for living—we can only survive a few days without it. We included it in the Nutrition Countdown because it often gets overlooked. The need for getting plenty of fluids is no secret, but many of our clients wind up short in this department. The traditional eight 8-ounce servings of fluid a day is the same as drinking a half gallon (that's the size of your typical milk carton). We don't count beverages containing caffeine here (such as regular coffee and tea) because caffeine is a diuretic which pushes fluids out of the body—it's a wash. Other fluids, such as juice and milk, can help meet your water quota.

Meals. We've talked about how important it is to *make peace with food*. Here's a useful tool that extends this principle to nutrition for meals. Visualize your plate as a peace sign:

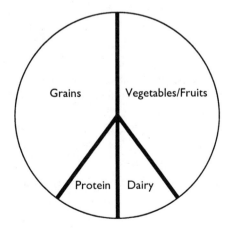

This serves two purposes: It gives you an easy-to-remember guide for healthy eating, and it helps to serve as a reminder to keep the peace with food.

So Where's the Chocolate?

As we said, we're not going to pull a fast one. There are no forbidden foods; deprivation doesn't work. All of the above guidelines are intended as a balance over time—which means even if you eat a candy bar, it will eventually average out. When you have let go of the diet mentality and have made peace with food, you will discover that you sometimes have a desire for food that has no nutritionally redemptive powers or clearly does not promote weight loss—*junk food*. Junk food is one of the most commonly used terms to describe what's considered unhealthy foods. But eating these types of foods doesn't mean you are an unhealthy eater. Here's a favorite story I (ER) like to tell that illustrates this point:

One day my son said to me, "Mom, what happens to people who don't eat as healthfully as you do?" His question sparked a sense of pride in me that, as a nutritionist, I had taught my son the virtues of healthy eating. My response to him included some lofty comments about how *those* people had a higher incidence of heart disease, diabetes, cancer, and so forth. But before I could get the words fully out of my mouth, he pointed to me with his best adolescent "Got you" finger and said, "But sometimes I see *you* eating chocolate and other junk foods!" I had to stop and laugh for a moment, and then said, "You're right, honey. Only 90 percent of what I eat is for my health, and 10 percent is for pleasure." I explained that just as my *play* time helps supply a vital balance to my life, those foods that he called junk gave me true satisfaction in my eating and so could be part of a balanced diet. From that point on, I have replaced the term "junk food" with "play food" for its role in the world of eating satisfaction.

But how can eating play foods be healthy? This is where you pull together all the intuitive eating skills, which means, in a nutshell, listening to your body. This is key. For example, if you were to eat chocolate all day long, there's a very good chance you would experience the following physical feelings: nausea, heaviness, dullness, and so forth. The question to you is, do you want to continue feeling this way? The truth is, if you listen to your body, it does not feel good eating this way. Even kids exposed to gobs of Halloween candy do not want to indulge for long. And when you know you can truly have the food again (chocolate, or whatever), it doesn't take much to satisfy you.

One client, Joe, was extremely fond of chocolate. He had truly made peace with food and was also at the stage of honoring his health. He was grocery shopping and discovered a new *triple* chocolate ice cream dessert, which was very rich. He chose not to buy it, not because it was loaded in fat, but because he did not want to experience what he calls headache food. He did not feel deprived; he knew he could have chocolate whenever he wished, and instead bought a few chocolate-covered raisins and was satisfied.

What About Fat?

Many people seem to think that eating healthfully means eating no fat at all. Contrary to popular belief, you do need some fat in your diet. *Fat is a nutrient*. Essential fatty acids are like vitamins in that your body cannot make them in adequate quantities, so you need them in your diet for health. There are two essential fatty acids, linolenic and linoleic acid. And if you don't get enough linoleic acid, your body doesn't make enough of another fatty acid, arachidonic acid. Therefore, arachidonic acid is considered an essential fatty acid when a linoleic acid deficiency exists. Consider some of the vital roles that fat plays in the body:

- It's a component of every cell membrane in the body.
- It helps to absorb the fat-soluble vitamins, A, D, E, and K.
- It helps maintain health of skin and hair.
- The brain and retina especially need linolenic acid.
- It helps to make hormones.

It is true, however, that too much fat in the diet is related to many chronic diseases, including heart disease and cancer. Health organizations from the government to the American Heart Association recommend getting no more than 30 percent of your calories from fat. But this does not mean that you need to be on a fat-free diet to be healthy or to achieve a healthy weight. The low-fat message has been taken to extreme levels for many chronic dieters, and has created the fat-free trap.

The Fat-Free Trap. Because fat has become the national enemy, it has spawned a profitable cottage industry of fat-free foods—from fat-free cheese to fat-free potato chips and ice cream. While this may seem advantageous to the American diet, we've seen problems, especially for chronic dieters.

One of the most common problems we see is the idea that "it doesn't count, I can eat as much as I want." The problem with this thinking is that it can actually lead to overeating. Instead of responding to satiety levels, it often becomes an affair of "I'm going to eat it all." When inner satiety cues are bypassed, it provokes a further dissonance from your body. In addition, *fat-free does not mean calorie-free*. A loaf of fat-free chocolate cake can easily have 1,000 calories. Ironically, many of our clients discover that if they were to have the real version of a food, they'd end up eating much less and therefore eat fewer calories, because since the real food is more satisfying, they would remain in touch with satiety cues.

Eating fat-free foods is *not* the epitomy of healthy eating. Sugar is naturally fat-free, yet one would hardly want to base a diet on sugar for health. Yet that's what many people are doing when they build diets based primarily on processed fat-free foods. Many of the fat-free products are high in sugar (especially the desserts) and low in whole grains. For example, Rice Krispies cereal proclaims on its label that it's always been fat-free. But it's also always been low in fiber. This type of fat-free eating is often nothing more than what we call the white bread diet—low in vitamin E (a valuable antioxidant), low in fiber, and low in other nutrients. If your prime mission in eating is selecting processed fat-free foods, you could easily end up with a nutritionally weak diet. There's nothing wrong with eating fat-free foods as an adjunct to a healthy diet. But you cannot assume that just because you've been eating 100 percent fat-free foods your diet is healthy.

How to Balance the Fat. So how do you keep your fat to a healthy level—respecting both your palate and the health of your body? If low-fat eating is pursued in a deprivational manner, it can be short-lived like any other diet. This was clearly illustrated in a follow-up study of the Women's Health Trial (WHT). The study examined factors that influenced a woman's ability to maintain a low-fat diet. These women (525 subjects) had been on a low-fat diet as a component of the WHT for at least one year. The researchers concluded that with respect to food choices, "the single strongest deterrent to maintaining a low-fat diet was the feeling of deprivation." Keep in mind that the purpose of this study was not to lose weight, but to see if a low-fat diet would reduce the risk of breast cancer.

There are three principles to consider when managing your fat intake:

1. *Discover how you can cut the fat without missing it or feeling deprived.* For example, most people can't tell the difference between whole milk and low-fat milk, so it's easy to make a switch which honors both your taste buds and palate. While many of our clients complain that they can't stand the "blue stuff," skim milk can easily be used in cooking without detection. Here are some other examples of how you might be able to cut the fat without missing it:

- Substitute applesauce for oil in cakes and baked goods.
- Use no-stick vegetable spray for cooking rather than oil.
- Try jam instead of butter on toast.
- Choose low-fat or nonfat dairy products.

2. *When possible, choose healthier fats.* Healthier fats are the ones lowest in saturated fatty acids. Saturated fats raise blood cholesterol and are found primarily in animal products such as meat, butter, and full fat dairy products. Saturated fats are also found in tropical oils such as coconut oil and palm oil. The oils lowest in saturated fats are: canola, corn, olive, safflower, and sunflower. Healthier fats can also be found in fatty fish such as salmon, as well as in avocado, most nuts, and seeds.

3. *When you eat fat, make sure it's worth it.* If I'm going to eat fat, I want to taste it! Many times food can be loaded with fat when it's not necessary, even redundant. For example, a tuna salad sandwich often has mayonnaise in both the tuna mixture and on the bread. Not only is that superfluous, you can't even taste the difference! Yet, a few teaspoons of olive oil drizzled on a pasta dish might

make all the difference in blending flavors. (At the same time, it's not necessary to drown the pasta dish in oil.) Or, adding toasted almonds adds a special flavor, texture, and aroma to many dishes.

Is There Anything Wrong with Counting Fat Grams? Being aware of fat grams can be very helpful to your health. But if you are militant about monitoring fat grams, it may just be masking an underlying diet mentality. Becoming aware of fat grams can help in:

• Food product comparison. If two products have similar taste but one is lower in fat grams, then by all means choose the lower fat product. Using fat grams in this manner helps to honor both your palate and your health.

• Informed food choices. When you have a general sense of the fat content of foods it may help guide your eating decisions. Suppose you discover for the first time that cheese has nine grams of fat per ounce. If cheese has been a food that you could take or leave, you may decide it's not worth the fat, because you don't enjoy it that much. So when eating out you might opt to hold the cheese, and instead, eat lower fat cheeses when at home.

HOW TO KEEP THE PLEASURE
IN HEALTHY EATING

If we are to change our eating attitudes to enlightened hedonism, we need to balance information with the pleasure of eating. The information part comes from two sources, listening to your body and the nutrition guidelines we presented earlier in the chapter. Listening to your body means not only staying in touch with satiety levels, but assessing the following questions:

• Do I really like the taste of these foods, or am I being a diet/health martyr?
• How does this food or type of meal make my body feel? Do I like this feeling?
• How do I feel when eating consistently in this manner? Do I like this feeling?
• Am I experiencing differences in my energy level?

If eating healthfully is a pleasurable experience *and* makes you feel better, you are more likely to continue honoring your health with your food choices. The key, however is not to turn the idea of healthy eating into an all-or-nothing prospect based on deprivation. Deprivation does not work in the long run.

Do savor your food. If you feel inclined to eat a fatty dessert or meal, make it a time when you can truly enjoy the food experience. Doing it while closing a business deal or driving a car usually will not be ideal because you will be preoccupied. You may be left wanting. Author Geneen Roth aptly compares this type of eating to daydreaming while engaged in a conversation. Even though you are physically present, you don't experience the words. ". . . the sense of being somewhere but not really being there, the 'sorry, how's that again?' feeling. . . . The conversation or event took place, but because attention wasn't present, it didn't take place for us, in us."

We might take a lesson from the French in the art of savoring the meal—and doing so could help our health. The French have a greater life expectancy and fewer deaths from cardiovascular disease than Americans, in spite of eating a diet that appears to be higher in fat—the highly publicized French paradox. Less publicized, but just as important, the French have fewer eating disorders and aren't dieting as much as Americans. While it has been speculated that wine consumption may explain the paradox, we believe it could be the relationship that the French have with food. The French have a more positive attitude toward food; it's viewed as one of life's pleasures, not as poison. They look forward to their meals and spend more time eating them. Ironically, our clients who have traveled to France describe how much they enjoyed the eating experience, the celebration of food without the worry—*they had discovered this even before working with the Intuitive Eating process.*

DON'T LET YOURSELF BE PUT ON A FOOD PEDESTAL

At first our clients think we must be perfect in our eating habits; after all, we are nutritionists. We are not food and nutrition goddesses and do not want to be placed on a pedestal. Some of the best information we've passed on to our patients is not about how nutritiously we

FRANCE VERSUS THE UNITED STATES:
DIETING AND LOW-CALORIE AND REDUCED-FAT FOODS*

	France	United States
Incidence of dieting (% of total population)	16%	26%
Use of low-calorie and reduced-fat foods and beverages (% of total population)	48%	76%
Consumption of low-fat products (% of total population)	39%	68%

*Adapted from Calorie Control Council National Surveys. *Calorie Control Commentary* 14 (1):1–2 (1992).

eat, but rather that we ate a whole piece of tiramisu and enjoyed each bite. Or how we got stuck with our food down, so to speak, and gobbled the nearest candy bar. And in spite of these times, we balance out our nutrition. We still honor our health, and our taste buds, and our humanness.

Many of our clients have been elevated to a place of specialness among their friends, colleagues, and family members because they *appear* to eat so well. "She is the health-conscious one." While in the beginning it's fun to garner the extra attention, after a while most of our clients do not want this notoriety. It adds pressure. When you are on this food pedestal it can intensify feelings of deprivation. It often means sneaking around to eat, which doesn't feel good or creates fears of "getting caught." My goodness, to get caught "cheating" on your diet! Horrors!

Our clients usually feel relieved when they voluntarily dethrone themselves as food-fitness paragons. What this means is they no longer need to be closet eaters or to put on a false food face. If they feel like ordering dessert with a meal, they will. It's their opportunity to show how you don't have to be perfect to value health and fitness.

Epilogue

This may be the end of the book, but if you choose to become an Intuitive Eater, it becomes a new beginning.

Take the journey to becoming an Intuitive Eater, and you will go through a process that is bound to challenge some of your most entrenched thoughts, and perhaps stir up some deeply hidden feelings and fears. You know that living in a world of dieting chaos with its self-blame and failure doesn't work. It doesn't work metabolically or emotionally, and it certainly doesn't work spiritually. Clients talk over and over about feeling beaten down, defeated—as if their souls are actually hurting. By the time they come to this process, many have given up hope of ever being normal eaters.

But becoming an Intuitive Eater requires a highly conscious decision and commitment. It means letting go of the old way of surviving and opening up to a new way of viewing life. It might take soul searching and introspective work to decide whether dieting has been keeping you from your deepest appreciation of life. Making this viewpoint change can be difficult to accomplish initially, but can ultimately become a way of living that knows no return.

To begin this paradigm shift, you'll need to consider that there are many tradeoffs in the eating world. Having the "willpower" to stay on a diet can give you a temporary sense of power and control, but being an Intuitive Eater gives you a lifelong sense of self-empowerment. The acts of dieting and rebound bingeing can offer excitement. So does eating forbidden foods. But when excitement no longer comes from food or dieting, other aspects of life are free to be experienced. When you are using food or the obsession that dieting creates to numb yourself or to distract yourself from your feelings the majority of time, you might feel calmer and less stressed, but your life can seem like a blurred, out-of-focus home movie. You know you're alive and racing through life, but you rarely experience its highs, lows, and nuances of sensation. Once you peel off the layers of dieting and overeating numbness, you'll discover a richness in life that for some has been buried for decades.

When you become an Intuitive Eater who responds to those innate biological and food preference signals, you get in touch with your body, thoughts, and feelings. Ultimately, this sensitivity can change the rest of your life.

You also learn to operate out of curiosity rather than judgment. When dieting, every digression from the food plan becomes an opportunity to become critical of yourself. And criticism can be deadly and infectious. It's not unusual for this critical viewpoint to spill over into other behaviors or even to family members and friends. As an Intuitive Eater, you see the food experience as an opportunity to learn more about your thoughts and feelings. You may find that this curiosity triggers other explorations in your life. You may even decide to make serious changes in other parts of your life that have been making you stressed or unhappy. Some clients have decided to change jobs or remove themselves from abusive relationships as a result of going deeper into the meaning of life. Others decide to get into counseling with a therapist.

One of our clients aptly suggested that Intuitive Eating is about *waiting* and learning to be patient. She finds herself *waiting* to eat until she is hungry. Then she describes *waiting* during a time-out in the midst of her meal to see if she is full. When she is experiencing a difficult feeling that she used to cover up with overeating, she now sits with the feeling and *waits* it out until she feels better. And in the bigger picture, she is *waiting* for her eating to normalize so that her body will return to its natural healthy weight. She says that this process has taught her to be more patient than she has ever been in her life. She has decided that patience is golden, that what she has learned about herself as she patiently *waits* is more valuable than all the pounds she has lost (and, of course, regained) and all the money she has spent on her failed diets. Learning to *wait* has freed her from the burden of dieting and from a life she felt locked into, with no escape.

We deeply hope that you will be able to free yourself from dieting by reclaiming the Intuitive Eating ability with which you were born.

Appendix

Common Questions and Answers About Intuitive Eating

We have compiled some of the questions most frequently asked by our clients as they go through the process of Intuitive Eating. We hope that these answers will also be answers to some of your questions.

Question #1: How long will this process take?
Answer: Unfortunately, this question has no pat answer. It depends on how long you've been dieting and how entrenched the voices of the Food Police are. It also depends on how willing you are to put weight loss off and concentrate on changing your relationship with food. We have seen some people connect quite rapidly with the concept and take only a month or two to be eating in a new way. For others, it's taken much longer to accept the principles and make serious changes.

Question #2: If I let myself eat whatever I want, won't I eat uncontrollably and gain lots of weight?
Answer: When you have made complete peace with food and know that what you like will always be available to you, you'll be able to stop after a moderate amount. If you're only giving yourself pseudo-permission, it won't work, because you don't really believe you'll always have access to this food. So check out how genuine your permission-giving is. Remember, guilt is what tends to make people

eat uncontrollably. Intuitive Eating means having no guilt in your eating.

Question #3: Won't my friends be judgmental and question my eating?

Answer: You may find that many people won't understand what you're doing. Most of our society is conditioned to dieting as the only means of losing weight or maintaining weight. In fact, some people are perpetually talking about being on diets or saying that they should be on diets. So, yes, some people will be judgmental. You may find that it's hard to explain what you are doing. Remember, this is an intuitive process. Some of the time, you'll just be feeling your way through it, knowing that it feels right.

Question #4: Should I try to explain what I'm doing?

Answer: You can try, but it might be frustrating. Key phrases to give out would be:

- Dieting leads to deprivation, deprivation leads to craving, and craving can lead to out-of-control behavior.
- I eat whatever I want when I'm hungry and find that I'm more easily able to stop when I'm full.
- When I feel satisfied with what I eat, I eat less.
- I'm learning to cope with my emotions without using food.

Question #5: Will I ever lose weight doing this?

Answer: It depends on your *natural healthy weight*—the weight your body will maintain with *normal* eating and *normal* exercise. If you've fluctuated between periods of dieting and overeating, you can probably reach your natural healthy weight. If you've used food to cope emotionally, you can reach your natural healthy weight. But if you're already at your natural healthy weight and have an unrealistic view of what you should weigh and are trying to be even thinner, you won't lose weight through Intuitive Eating. Also, for some people, their metabolism has been altered and damaged by years of excessive dieting and weight yo-yos. For them, extra exercise combined with gradually increasing the food they eat might be the only means for speeding up the metabolism and getting some of the extra weight off.

Question #6: What if I can't lose weight? What's this all worth?
Answer: If you are someone who is genetically destined to weigh more than society's standards and therefore cannot lose weight, you will derive a great deal of peace and contentment with this process. You will get off the "treadmill" of deprivation and guilt. You will eat in a way that's pleasurable and satisfying. You will stop feeling guilty about your eating and stop blaming yourself for being over-weight. You will stop overeating and with that stop feeling bloated and uncomfortable. You'll stop intermittently undereating and with that stop feeling starved and uncomfortable. Achieving an intuitive eating style will free your time for more enriching thoughts and feelings (rather than food-worry and guilt). For many people, that means ultimately feeling happier.

Question #7: What if I never feel hungry?
Answer: Some people report that they don't feel hunger in their stomachs, but get raging headaches or some other symptom from not having eaten. For some people, they've dieted and/or binged for so long that they've lost complete touch with hunger. If this is the case for you, you can give yourself a period of time where you purposely eat every three to four hours to try to reestablish your hunger signals. Your body needs food in these intervals, and you may find that after a while your body trusts it's going to get fed and will respond by expressing hunger.

Question #8: How will I know when I'm full?
Answer: When you have learned to *honor your hunger*, you'll find that your fullness signals are much more apparent to you. If you eat all of the time and don't feel hunger, it's hard to experience fullness. You'll have no base with which to start to judge the difference. It's helpful to take a time-out in the middle of your meal to test your fullness.

Question #9: Can I ever eat something if it just looks good, but I'm not hungry?

Answer: The Intuitive Eating process is not another diet with a set of absolute rules. Although *honoring your hunger* is one of the first principles, there will be many times when you'll choose to eat something just for its taste or sensual pleasure, without being hungry. We call this taste hunger. If you give yourself permission for occasional responses to taste hunger, you'll feel more satisfied with your entire eating experience and find that you end up eating smaller quantities of food in general.

Question #10: What about sweets? Should I eat them when I'm hungry?

Answer: In general, if you wait until you're hungry to eat sweets, you'll find that you may end up eating a larger quantity than you might need to satisfy your sweet tooth, because you'll be trying to satisfy your biological hunger. Most cultures offer sweets at the end of the meal to please the palate. Having something sweet at that point is usually in response to taste hunger.

Question #11: What if I want to eat when I can't handle my feelings?

Answer: Generally, the quickest route to resolving emotional conflict is to allow yourself to experience your feelings to their utmost. But sometimes this can be overwhelming. Some people need to be with a friend or a therapist to feel safe enough to let their feelings come out. Others are able to tolerate their feelings for some period of time, but then need an escape for a while until they feel able to deal with them again. If that is where you find yourself, then search for healthy ways to comfort and distract yourself from the feelings so that you don't end up diving into food as a way of coping.

Question #12: What about good nutrition? If I eat whatever I like, won't I be unhealthy?

Answer: We have found, in case after case, that giving yourself permission to eat whatever you like ultimately results in a 90–10 balance of food choice. You'll find, after you have finally made peace with food, that about 90 percent of your food choices will be fairly light and nutritionally healthy and 10 percent will be play food. The 90 percent healthy takes care of your body while the 10 percent play takes care of your soul! After all, if you never have to be deprived of a favorite food again, you won't have a great urge to overdo on it. You'll want to feel good, and feeling good comes from eating lightly without stuffing yourself.

Question #13: Do I have to exercise to make this work?

Answer: We have put our chapter on exercise toward the end of the book, because we find that too much emphasis on exercise in the beginning of this process can make some people feel as if they're on another diet. Exercise is something that you'll probably want to do because it makes you feel good. If you disconnect your eating from your exercise, you'll find that you don't get into the old trap of feeling that exercise is for the purpose of weight loss. Exercise is a benefit for all people, young or old, slim or overweight. It's part of a healthy existence. If you are someone who is adamant about not exercising, the Intuitive Eating process will still be of benefit to you, because it frees you from the world of dieting. But wait and see, you may find yourself exercising despite yourself!

Question #14: Should I tell others that they should try Intuitive Eating?

Answer: Most people don't like being told what to do. It usually makes them feel rebellious. You're probably better off just living this new lifestyle. If people ask you why you seem so calm and nonobsessed about food or why you look so radiant, you can tell them what you're doing. They might then ask about doing it themselves.

Question #15: What do I do if a host or hostess tries to push more food on me when I don't want anymore?

Answer: This person is not respecting your boundaries and does not have a right to pressure you. Say "No, thank you" firmly. Say that you're full and don't want to feel uncomfortable. Remember, your intuitive signals are what count, and you need to honor them.

References

Chapter 1. Hitting Diet Bottom

Associated Press. Long Decline in U.S. Smoking Ends. *Orange County Register*, California, April 2, 1993.

Levine, S. Smoke Yourself Thin. *On the Issues* Summer (1994):29–31.

Wiseman, C., et al. Increasing pressure to be thin: 19 years of diet products in television commercials. *Eating Disorders: The Journal of Treatment and Prevention* 1, 1(1993):55.

Chapter 2. What Kind of Eater Are You?

Berg, F. *The Health Risks of Weight Loss*. Hettinger, N. D.: Healthy Living Institute, 1993.

Birch, L. L. Children's eating: Are manners enough? *Journal of Gastronomy* 7, 1(1993):19–25.

———. The role of experience in children's food acceptance patterns. *Journal of the American Dietetic Association* 87, 9 supplement (1987):5–36.

Birch, L. L., Johnson, S. L., Andresen, G., Peters, J. C., and Schulte, M. C. The variability of young children's energy intake. *New England Journal of Medicine* 324(1991):232.

Eating guilt. *Obesity and Health* 6, 2(1992):43.

Forbes, G. B. Children and Food—Order Amid Chaos. *New England Journal of Medicine* 324(1991):262.

Gallup Organization. Gallup Survey of Public Opinion Regarding Diet and Health. Prepared for American Dietetic Association/International Food Information Council. Princeton, N. J.: Gallup Organization, January 1990.

Hill, A. J., and Robinson, A. Dieting concerns have a functional effect on the behaviour of nine-year-old girls. *British Journal of Clinical Psychology* 30 (1991):265–67.

Satter, E. Comments from a practitioner on Leann Birch's research. *Journal of the American Dietetic Association* 87, 9 supplement (1987):5-41.

———. *How to Get Your Child to Eat . . . But Not Too Much.* Palo Alto, Calif.: Bull Publishing, 1987, p. 6.

Warning: Keep Dieting Out of Reach of Children. *Tufts University Diet & Nutrition Letter* 11, 10(1993):3.

Chapter 5. Principle 1: Reject the Diet Mentality

Associated Press (Washington). Vitamin retailer to pay fine. *AP Online*, April 29, 1994.

Berdanier, C. D., and McIntosh, M. K. Weight loss—weight regain: A vicious cycle. *Nutrition Today* 26, 5(1991):6.

Berg, F. M. *The Health Risks of Weight Loss.* Hettinger, N. D.: Healthy Living Institute, 1993.

Blackburn, G. L., et al. Weight cycling: The experience of human dieters. *American Journal of Clinical Nutrition* 49(1989):1105.

———. Why and how to stop weight cycling in overweight adults. *Eating Disorders Review* 4, 1(1993):1.

Ciliska, D. *Beyond Dieting.* New York, N.Y.: Brunner/Mazel, 1990.

Foreyt, J. P., and Goodrick, G. K. *Living Without Dieting.* Houston, Tx.: Harrison, 1992.

———. Weight Management Without Dieting. *Nutrition Today* March/April (1993):4.

Gallup Organization. Women's Knowledge and Behavior Regarding Health and Fitness. Conducted for American Dietetic Association and Weight Watchers, June 1993.

Garrow, J. S. Treatment of obesity. *Lancet* 340(1992):409–13.

Goodrick, G. K., and Foreyt, J. P. Why treatments for obesity don't last. *Journal of the American Dietetic Association* 91, 10(1991):1243.

Grodner, M. Forever dieting: Chronic dieting syndrome. *Journal of Nutrition Education* 24, 4(1992):207–10.

Hartmann, E. *Boundaries in the Mind. A New Psychology of Personality.* New York, N.Y.: Basic Books, 1991.

Hill, A. J., and Robinson, A. Dieting concerns have a functional effect on the behaviour of nine-year-old girls. *British Journal of Clinical Psychology* 30(1991):265–67.

Katherine, A. *Boundaries—Where You End and I Begin*. Park Ridge, Ill.: Parkside Publishing, 1991.

Kern, P. A., et al. The effects of weight loss on the activity and expression of adipose-tissue lipoprotein lipase in very obese humans. *New England Journal of Medicine* 322, 15(1990):1053–59.

National Research Council. *Diet and Health*. National Academy Press, Washington, D.C., 1989.

Polivy, J., and Herman, C. P. Undieting: A program to help people stop dieting. *International Journal of Eating Disorders* 11, 3(1992):261–68.

Rodin, J., et al. Weight cycling and fat distribution. *International Journal of Obesity* 14(1990):303–10.

Wilson, G. T. Short-Term Psychological Benefits and Adverse Effects of Weight Loss. NIH Technology Assessment Conference: Methods for Voluntary Weight Loss and Control, March 30–April 1, 1992.

Wooley S. C., and Garner, D. M. Obesity treatment: The high cost of false hope. *Journal of the American Dietetic Association* 91, 10(1991):1248.

Yanovski, S. Z. Are anorectic agents the magic bullet for obesity? Editorial. *Arch Family Medicine* 2(1993)1025–27.

Chapter 6. Principle 2: Honor Your Hunger

Birch, L. L., Johnson, S. L., Andresen, G., Peters, J. C., and Schulte, M. C. The variability of young children's energy intake. *New England Journal of Medicine* 324(1991):232.

Boyle, M. A., and Zyla, G. *Personal Nutrition*, 2nd ed. St. Paul, Minn.: West Publishing Co., 1992, pp. 77, 217.

Drott, C., and Lundholm, K. Cardiac effects of caloric restriction mechanisms and potential hazards. *International Journal Obesity* 16(1992):481–86.

Franchina, J. J., and Slank, K. L. Effects of deprivation on salivary flow in the apparent absence of food stimuli. *Appetite* 10(1988):143–47.

Garner, D. M., and Garfinkel, P. E. (eds). *Handbook of Psychotherapy for Anorexia and Bulimia* (chapter 21). New York, N.Y.: Guilford, 1985.

Leibowitz, S. Brain neuropeptide Y: An integrator of endocrine, metabolic and behavioral processes. *Brain Research Bulletin* 27(3–4)(1991):33–7.

Marano, H. Chemistry and craving. *Psychology Today* Jan.–Feb. (1993):31.

Nicolaidis, S., and Even, P. The metabolic signal of hunger and satiety, and its pharmacological manipulation. *International Journal of Obesity* 16, supplement 3(1992):531–41.

Polivy, J., and Herman, C. P. Diagnosis and treatment of normal eating. *Journal of Consulting and Clinical Psychology* 55, 5(1987):635–44.

――――. Dieting and bingeing, a causal analysis. *American Psychologist* Feb. (1985):193–201.

Scrimshaw, N. S. The phenomenon of famine. *Annual Review of Nutrition* 7(1987):1–21.

Wolf, N. *The Beauty Myth.* New York, N.Y.: Anchor, 1991, pp. 179–217.

Chapter 7. Principle 3: Make Peace with Food

Baldwin, A. L. *Theories of Child Development,* 2nd ed. New York, N.Y.: John Wiley, 1980.

Berk, L. E. *Child Development,* 3rd ed. Boston, Mass.: Allyn & Bacon, 1994.

Erikson, E. H. *The Life Cycle Completed: A Review.* New York, N.Y.: W. W. Norton, 1982.

Herman, C. P., and Polivy, J. Restrained Eating. In Stunkard, A. *Obesity.* Philadelphia, Pa.: W. B. Saunders Co., 1980, pp. 208–225.

Larson, Ennette, M. S., R. D. Personal communication. Research dietitian for NIH, Phoenix, Ariz., May 25, 1994.

Loro, A. D., and Orleans, C. S. Binge eating in obesity: Preliminary findings and guidelines for behavioral analysis and treatment. *Addictive Behaviours* 7(1981):155–66.

Miller, P.H. *Theories of Developmental Psychology.* New York, N.Y.: W. H. Freeman, 1993.

Mydans, S. 8 bid farewell to the future: Musty air, roaches and ants. *New York Times,* Sept. 27, 1993, p. A1.

Ogden, J., and Wardle, J. Cognitive and emotional responses to food. *International Journal of Eating Disorders* 10, 3(1991):297–311.

Satter, E. *How to Get Your Kid to Eat ... But Not Too Much.* Palo Alto, Calif.: Bull Publishing, 1987.

Seamon, J. G., and Kenrick, D. T. *Psychology,* 2nd ed. Englewood Cliffs, NJ: Prentice-Hall, 1994.

Chapter 8. Principle 4: Challenge the Food Police

As the Chicken Turns. *Tufts University Diet and Nutrition Letter* 11, 11(1994):1.

Berne, E. *Games People Play.* New York, N.Y.: Grove Press, 1964.

Ellis, A., and Harper, R. A. *A New Guide to Rational Living.* North Hollywood, Calif.: Wilshire Book Company, 1975.

Food Guilt. *Utne Reader* Nov.–Dec. 1993, p. 53–67.

Hiser, E. Butter paroled, margarine charged. *Eating Well* Nov.–Dec. (1993):104.

King, G. A., Herman, C. P., and Polivy, J. Food perception in dieters and non-dieters. *Appetite* 8(1987):147–58.

Seid, R. P. *Never Too Thin.* New York, N.Y.: Prentice-Hall, 1989.

Chapter 9. Principle 5: Feel Your Fullness

Bray, G. A. The nutrient balance approach to obesity. *Nutrition Today* 28, 3(1993):13–18.

De Castro, J. M. Physiological, environmental, and subjective determinants of food intake in humans: A meal pattern analysis. *Physiology & Behavior* 44(1988):651–59.

————. Weekly rhythms of spontaneous nutrient intake and meal patterns of humans. *Physiology & Behavior* 50(1991):729–38.

Chapter 10. Principle 6: Discover the Satisfaction Factor

Anderson, S. L. A look at the Japanese dietary guidelines. *Journal of the American Dietetic Association* 90, 11(1990):1527–28.

Visser, M. On having cake and eating it. *Journal of Gastronomy* 7, 1(1993):5–17.

Wisniewski, L., Epstein, L. H., and Caggiula, A.R. Effect of food change on consumption, hedonics, and salivation. *Physiology and Behavior* 92, 52(1992):21–26.

Chapter 11. Principle 7: Cope with Your Emotions Without Using Food

Arnow, B., Kenardy, J., and Agras, W. S. Binge eating among the obese: A descriptive study. *Journal of Behavioral Medicine* 15, 2(1992): 155–70.

Barnett, R. Appetite and the meal. *The Journal of Gastronomy* 7, 1(1993): 59–72.

Boyle, M. A., and Zyla, G. Personal Nutrition, 2nd ed. St. Paul, Minnesota: West Publishing Co., 1992, p. 214.

De Castro, J. M., and Brewer, E. M. The amount eaten in meals by humans is a power function of the number of people present. *Physiology and Behavior* 51(1991):121–25.

De Castro, J. M. Social facilitation of duration and size but not rate of the spontaneous meal intake of humans. *Physiology and Behavior* 47(1990): 1129–35.

————. Weekly rhythms of spontaneous nutrient intake and meal pattern of humans. *Physiology and Behavior* 50(1991):729–38.

Goldman, S. J., Herman, C. P., and Polivy, J. Is the effect of a social model on eating attenuated by hunger? *Appetite* 17(1991):129–40.

Heatherton, T. F., Herman, C. P., and Polivy, J. Effects of distress on eating: The importance of ego-involvement. *Journal of Personality and Social Psychology* 62, 5(1992):801–3.

Herman, C. P., and Polivy, J. Psychological factors in the control of appetite. *Current Concepts in Nutrition* 16(1988):41–51.

Herman, C. P., Polivy, J., Lank, C. N., and Heatherton, T. F. Anxiety, hunger, and eating behavior. *Journal of Abnormal Psychology* 96, 3(1987):264–69.

Hill, A. J., Weaver, C. F. L., and Blundell, J. E. Food craving, dietary restraint and mood. *Appetite* 17(1991):187–97.

Morton, C. J. Weight loss maintenance and relapse prevention. In Frankle, R. T., and Yang, M. *Obesity and Weight Control.* Rockville, MD: Aspen Publishers, 1988.

Ogden, J., and Wardle, J. Cognitive and emotional responses to food. *International Journal of Eating Disorders* 10, 3(1991):297–311.

Polivy, J., Herman, C. P., Hackett, R., and Kuleshnyk, I. The effects of self-attention and public attention on eating in restrained and unrestrained subjects. *Journal of Personality and Social Psychology* 50, 6(1986):1253–60.

Weissenburger, J., Rush, A. J., Giles, D. E., and Stunkard, A. J. Weight change in depression. *Psychiatry Research* 17(1986):275–83.

Chapter 12. Principle 8: Respect Your Body

Diet Winners and Sinners of the Year. *People Weekly.* January 10, 1994.

Oral communication with Elite Modeling Agency. New York, N.Y., Sept. 6, 1994.

Rodin, J. *Body Traps.* New York, N.Y.: William Morrow, 1992.

United States Department of Health and Human Services (USDHH). Dietary Guidelines for Americans, 3rd ed. Home and Garden Bulletin, no. 232, 1990.

Wiseman et al. Cultural expectations of thinness in women: An update. *International Journal of Eating Disorders* 11, 1(1992):85–89.

Chapter 13. Principle 9: Exercise—Feel the Difference

American College of Sports Medicine. Position Stand: The recommended quantity and quality of exercise for developing and maintaining cardiorespiratory and muscular fitness in healthy adults. *Medicine and Science in Sports and Exercise* 22(1990):265–74.

American College of Sports Medicine. Press release: Experts Release New Recommendations to Fight America's Epidemic of Physical Inactivity, July 29, 1993.

Evans, B., and Rosenberg, I. *Biomarkers: The 10 Determinants of Aging You Can Control.* New York, N.Y.: Simon & Schuster, 1991.

Foreyt, J. P., et al. Response of free-living adults to behavioral treatment of obesity: Attrition and compliance to exercise. *Behavior Therapy* 24 (1993):659–69.

Gavin, J. *The Exercise Habit.* Champaign, Ill.: Human Kinetics, 1992.

Lemon, P. W. R., and Mullin, J. P. Effect of initial muscle glycogen levels on protein catabolism during exercise. *Journal Applied Physiology: Respitr. Environ. Exercise Physiol.* 48, 4(1980):624–29.

Miller, W. C. Exercise: Americans don't think it's worth it. *Obesity & Health* Mar.–Apr. (1994):29.

Pollock, M. L., et al. Effect of age and training on aerobic capacity and body composition of master athletes. *Journal of Applied Physiology* 62 (1987):725–31.

Tryon, W. W., Goldberg, J. L., and Morrison, D. F. Activity decreases as percentage overweight increases. *International Journal of Obesity* 16 (1992):591–95.

Chapter 14. Principle 10: Honor Your Health—Gentle Nutrition

Callaway, W. The marriage of taste and health: A union whose time has come. *Nutrition Today* 27, 3(1992):37–42.

Glore, S. R., et al. Soluble fiber and serum lipids: A literature review. *Journal of the American Dietetic Association* 94(1994):425–36.

Ledoux, S. Eating disorders among adolescents in an unselected French population. *International Journal of Eating Disorders* 10, 1(1991):81–89.

McCargar, L. J., et al. Physiological effects of weight cycling in female lightweight rowers. *Canadian Journal of Applied Physiology* 18, 3(1993): 291–303.

National Research Council. *Recommended Dietary Allowances.* Washington, D.C.: National Academy of Sciences, 1989, pp. 46–49.

Roth, G. *Breaking Free from Compulsive Eating*. New York, N.Y.: Bobbs-Merrill, 1984, p. 37.

Rozin, P. Food and cuisine: Education, risk and pleasure. *Journal of Gastronomy* 7, 1(1993):111–20.

Schardt, D. Phytochemicals: Plants against cancer. *Nutrition Action Health Letter* 21, 3(1994):1.

Stacey, M. *Consumed: Why Americans Love Hate And Fear Food*. New York, N.Y.: Simon & Schuster, 1994.

Urban, N., et al. Correlates of maintenance of a low-fat diet among women in the women's health trial. *Preventive Medicine* 21(1992):279–91.

USDA. Human Nutrition Service. *USDA's Food Guide Pyramid*. Home and Garden Bulletin, no. 249, April 1992.

USDHH. Healthy People 2000. *Nutrition Today* 25, 6(1990):29–39.

Index

Absolutist thinking, 117
"air food," beware of, 132
American College of Sports Medicine
    (ACSM), 187–8
American Council on Exercise
    (ACE), 187
American Dietetic Association, 19, 196
American Heart Association, 207
American Institute of Wine & Food
    (AIWF), 187
*American Journal of Clinical
    Nutrition*, 195
Anorexia nervosa, 4, 12, 177
Antioxidants, 201
Anxiety, using food to relieve, 155
ATP, 68–9

Beans, as part of the diet, 204
Beauty Myth, The, 63
Berne, Eric, 97–8
Binge eating, xv, 2, 11, 12, 13, 44, 50,
    51, 66, 78–9, 113, 213
    see also Eating disorders
Biological hunger vs. emotional
    hunger, 38, 71–5, 77, 149–51,
    154–5
"Biological indifference," 70
Biological mechanisms that trigger
    eating, 64–70, 77
    carbohydrate craver—
        Neuropeptide Y, 65–6

heightened digestion, 65
powerhouse cell theory, 68–9
second-guessing your biology,
    69–70
Biosphere 2 experiment, 76, 77
Birch, Leann, 14–15
Body image obsessions and
    negativity, 1, 27–8, 35, 164–76
    rebuilding, 38, 39
    see also Body respect
Body respect, 168–76
    be realistic, 176
    change your body-assessment
        tools, 170
    don't compromise for the "Big
        Event," 172–4
    quit the body-check game, 170–2
    respect body diversity, 175–6
    stop body-bashing, 174–5
Body sculpting, 164–5
Body Traps, 166–7
Boredom eating, 152
Boundary Model for the Regulation
    of Eating, 69–70
Bribery and reward eating, 152–3
British Columbia, University of, 198
Bulimia, 4, 12, 62, 171

Caffeine abuse, as diet management
    tool, 4
California Daily Food Guide, 204

Cancer and its relationship to diet, 200, 201, 204, 206, 207
Captivity behavior, 81
Carbohydrates, 132–3
  essential carbohydrate power, 182
  importance of, 66–8
  Neuropeptide Y (NPY), 65–6
  preferred fuel, 181–3, 199–200
Careful Eater, 9, 10–11, 13, 16
  eating style, 10–11
  problem, 11
Catastrophic thinking, 118–19
Centers for Disease Control (CDC), 6, 187–8
Challenge the Food Police principle, 23–4
Chaotic Unconscious Eater, 9, 12, 16
Child, Julia, 197
Children:
  and dieting, problems of, 6–7, 17
  innate ability to regulate eating, 14–15
Chocolate and "junk foods," 206–7
Cholesterol:
  beans shown to lower blood, 204
  exercise increases good, and lowers total bad, 185
  medical referrals of patients with high, xiii
  soluble fiber role in lowering blood, 200
Chronic dieting, damage from, 49–51, 68
Comfort, using food as, 149–50
Conscious eating, 126–9
  Fullness Discovery Scale, 128
Consciousness, how to increase, 129–30
  defend yourself from Obligatory Eating, 130
  eat without distraction, 129
  reinforce your conscious decision to stop, 130

Consumed: Why Americans Love Hate and Fear Food, 195
Continuum of emotional eating, 149–51
  comfort, 149–50
  distraction, 149, 150
  punishment, 149, 151
  sedation, 149, 150–1
  sensory gratification, 149
Cope with your emotions without using food, principle, 26–7, 147–63
  continuum of emotional eating, 149–51
  coping with emotional eating, 156–7
  emotional triggers, 151–6
  how emotional eating has hurt *and* helped, 160–1
  using food constructively, 163
  when food is no longer important, 161–2
Costanzo, Philip, 15
Costill, David, 182
Couch-potato lifestyle, 186–7
Covey, Stephen, 48, 52
Cravings, food, 76–8
Crea, Joe, 18
Crystallization of Intuitive Eating style, 37–8

Dairy products, and the diet, 204–5
Depression era eating, 81–2
Depression, mild, and weight gain, 155
Diabetes, xiv, 185, 200, 206
Dichotomous thinking, 115–17
Diet backlash, 2–4, 84–6
Diet bonding, 42–3
Diet mentality, how to reject the, 48–60
  1. recognize and acknowledge the damage that dieting causes, 49–51

2. be aware of diet-mentality traits and thinking, 52–5

3. get rid of the dieter's tools, 55–9

Diet-mentality traits and thinking, 52–3
forget about failure, 55
forget being obedient, 53–5
forget willpower, 52–3

Diet Rebel, 98, 102–3, 106, 107, 108, 109, 110

Diet-type foods and products, 1, 12

Dieter's Dilemma, the, 47–8

Dieter's tools, get rid of the, 55–9

Dieting:
backlash as cumulative side effect of, 2, 84–6, 136
can't fight biology, 7
children and, 6–7, 14–15
crash, 183
damage from, 49–51
decreased sense of willpower and, 18
eat-healthful-or-die messages, 18–19
eating disorders and, 4, 17, 177
fear of not, 41–2, 88–92
food fundamentalism and eating morality, 95
guilt and, 1, 4, 21, 36, 84–6, 94–5
hitting diet bottom, 1–7
increased feelings of deprivation, 17
makes food the enemy, 1
myths, 111
paradox, 4–7
process of, 1–2
psychological and emotional damage from, 51
slows metabolism, 1, 17, 50
social withdrawal and, 3
triggers emotions that lead to using food to cope with feelings, 149

unconscious forms of, 8
yo-yo, 11

Digestion, heightened, 65

Discover the satisfaction factor, principle, 25–6, 134–46, 149
don't be afraid to enjoy your food, 136
how to regain your pleasure in eating, 137–46
it doesn't have to be perfect, 146
reclaim the right to pleasurable, satisfying eating, 146
wisdom of pleasure, 135–6

Distraction, using food as, 149, 150, 159–60

Eaters, types of, 8–18
see also specific types

Eating disorders, 4–5, 12, 177
see also specific disorders

Eating Disorders—The Journal of Treatment and Prevention, 4–5

Eating personalities, 9–19
Careful Eater, 9, 10–11, 13, 16
Intuitive Eater, 10, 17
Professional Dieter, 9, 11–12, 13, 17
Unconscious Eater, 9, 12–13, 16
when your personality works against you, 13–14

Eating voices, 98–107
Diet Rebel, 98, 102–3, 106, 107, 108, 109, 110
Food Anthropologist, 98, 103–5, 107, 108, 109
Food Police, 98–100, 105, 106, 107, 108, 110
how they emerge and evolve, 107–10
Nurturer, 105–6, 108, 109, 110
Nutrition Ally, 98, 99, 101, 102, 109, 110
Nutrition Informant, 98, 100–2, 106, 107, 108, 110
Rebel Ally, 98, 99, 106, 109, 110

Eating Well magazine, 95
Ego states, 97–8
Ellis, Albert, 111
Emotional hunger, 75, 147–9
  see also Cope with your emotions
  without using food
Emotional Unconscious Eater, 13, 17
Endurance athlete, 182–3
Erikson, Erik, 92
Even, P., 68–9
"Exchange system" for diabetic meal
  planning and weight control, xiv
Excitement of food when life feels
  dull, 153
Exercise—feel the difference,
  principle, 28–9, 40, 181–92
  abuse, 191
  be comfortable, 190
  breaking through the exercise
    barriers, 183–8
  don't get caught in exercise mind
    games, 185–8
  focus on how it feels, 184
  focus on it as a way of taking care
    of yourself, 185
  get active in daily living, 188–9
  getting started on a lifelong
    commitment, 188–90
  include strength training, 190
  make exercise fun, 189
  make exercise a nonnegotiable
    priority, 189
  remember rest, 191–2
Exploration and discovery stage to
  eating intuitively, 35–7

Fad diets, 1
Fat, and the diet, 207–10
Feel your fullness, principle, 24–5,
  39, 123–33
  fullness factors, 130–3
  how to respect your fullness,
    126–30
  key to respecting fullness, 125

recognizing comfortable satiety,
    125–6
  what if you can't stop eating?, 133
  what if you feel there's something
    missing?, 133
Feelings and situations that trigger
  desire to eat, 151–6
  anxiety, 155
  being connected, 155
  boredom and procrastination, 152
  bribery and reward, 152–3
  excitement, 153
  frustration, anger, and rage, 154
  loosening the reins, 155–6
  love, 154
  mild depression, 155
  soothing, 153–4
  stress, 154–5
Food Anthropologist, 98, 103–5, 107,
    108, 109, 121, 126
  keeping food journal, 104
Food deprivation, power of, 61–3,
    63–4
Food Police, xvi, 4, 98–100, 105, 106,
    107, 111
  challenge the, 23–4, 94–122
  food talk, 96–7
  self-awareness—the ultimate
    weapon against the, 121–2
  self-talk, 111–14
  who's talking, 97–107
Food Pyramid guidelines, 199
Foods with staying power, 132–3
Foreyt, John P., 2, 47, 48
France vs. U.S. in diet styles, 211–12
"Free foods," xiv
Fruits and vegetables, important to
  health, 200–2
Frustration and anger, using food to
  subdue, 154
Fullness Discovery Scale, 127, 128

Garner, David, 51
Glucose, importance of, 67–8

Goodrick, G. Ken, 47, 48
Grains, as fuel for body, 199–200
Grapefruit diet, 1, 76
Guilt and eating, 1, 4, 21, 36, 84–6,
  94–5

Habituation effect, 89
Harper, Robert A., 111
Harvard Alumni Health Study, 50
Harvard School of Public Health, 18
Heart disease risks of chronic
  dieting, 50–1, 68, 206
Hedonics and food, 145–6
Heider, Fritz, 77
Herman, C. Peter, 69–70, 82
High blood pressure, xiii, 185
Honor your health—gentle nutrition,
  principle, 29–30, 193–212
  don't let yourself be put on a food
    pedestal, 211–12
  how to keep pleasure in healthy
    eating, 210–11
  making peace with nutrition,
    196–8
  practicing gentle nutrition,
    198–210
  tenet of food wisdom, 195–6
  what is healthy eating?, 194–5
Honor your hunger, principle, 21–2,
  36–7, 38, 39–40, 61–70, 128
  how to honor biological hunger,
    71–5
  hunger silence, 71
  mechanisms that trigger eating,
    64–70
  primal food therapy, 70–1
  primal hunger, 63–4
Hunger Discovery Scale, 74, 127
Hunger silence, causes of, 71
  chaos, 71
  dieting, 71
  numbing, 71
  skipping breakfast, 71
Hyperconsciousness, 35–6, 37, 72

"Ideal" weight vs. natural healthy
  weight, 176–8
Intuitive Eater(s), 15–17, 106–7, 109,
  122, 148–9, 167, 171
  awakening the, through stages,
    31–40
  don't finish eating something you
    don't like, 144–5
  how your Intuitive Eater gets
    buried, 17–19
  journey to becoming, 213–15
  see also Intuitive Eating *and
    specific topics*
Intuitive Eating:
  development of process, xv,
    14–15, 31–40
  dieting vs., 32–4
  natural, 14–15
  questions and answers about,
    216–20
  tools, 60
  see also specific principles
Intuitive Eating, principles of, 20–30
  1. reject the diet mentality, 20–1,
    41–60
  2. honor your hunger, 21–2,
    61–75
  3. make peace with food, 22–3,
    76–93
  4. challenge the Food Police,
    23–4, 94–122
  5. feed your fullness, 24–5,
    123–33
  6. discover the satisfaction factor,
    25–6, 134–46
  7. cope with your emotions
    without using food, 26–7,
    147–63
  8. respect your body, 27–8,
    164–80
  9. exercise—feel the difference,
    28–9, 181–92
  10. honor your health—gentle
    nutrition, 29–30, 193–212

Intuitive Eating, stages of, 31–40
1. readiness—hitting diet bottom, 34–5
2. exploration, conscious learning and pursuit of pleasure, 35–7
3. crystallization, 37–8
4. the Intuitive Eater awakens, 38–9
5. final stages—treasure the pleasure, 39–40

Japanese, the, and healthy living, 25
Jenny Craig diet, 1
"Junk food," 206

Ketosis, 68
Keys, Ancel, 61, 63, 77

Last-Bite Threshold, 127–8
Last Supper eating, 3, 4, 11, 22, 76, 79–80
Laxatives, diuretics, and diet pills, 12
Linear thinking, 120–1
Liposuction, 7
Love through food, showing, 154

Make peace with food, principle, 22–3, 36, 38, 39, 76–95, 125, 206
deprivation backlash—rebound eating, 78–9
deprivation set-up, 77–8
how is dieting possible?, 82–6
the key—*unconditional* permission, 86–93
Maslow's Hierarchy of Needs, 64
Media pressure to diet, 5–6, 95
Medical problems of overweight, xiii–xv
Men's Fitness, 6
Men's Health, 6
Metabolism:
feed your, 199

increased, due to exercise, 185
sluggish, due to dieting, 3, 17, 50
Moss, Kate, 165

National Cancer Institute, 200
National Institutes of Health Weight Loss and Control Conference (1992), 51
Needs, meeting without food, 158–60
deal with your feelings, 159
find a different distractor, 159–60
seek nurture, 158–9
Negative self-talk and how to change it, 111, 113, 114–21
absolutist thinking, 117–18
catastrophic thinking, 118–19
dichotomous thinking, 115–17
linear thinking, 120–1
pessimistic thinking, or "the cup is half empty," 119–20
Neuropeptide Y (NPY), 65–6
Never Too Thin, 95
New England Journal of Medicine, 14
Nicolaidis, S., 68–9
Nurture, seek, instead of food, 158–9
Nurturer, 105–6, 108, 109, 110, 122
Nutrition, 29–30, 193–212
role of in preventing chronic disease, 193–4
tenets of good, 195–6
Nutrition Ally, 98, 99, 101, 102, 109, 110
Nutrition Countdown and nutritional guidelines, 199–206
Nutrition Informant, 98, 100–2, 106, 107, 108, 110, 121
Nutrition Labeling Education Act (NLEA), 194–5

Obesity and Health, 18
Obesity and overt prejudice, 176

Obligatory Eating, defend yourself from, 130
One-last-diet trap, the, 43–4
Optifast, 1
Osteoporosis, 204–5

Personal trainer and exercise program, 187
Pessimistic thinking, 119–20
Phytochemicals, 201
"Play foods," 206–7
Pleasure as a goal of healthy eating, 135–6
　1. ask yourself what you *really* want to eat, 137–8
　2. discover the pleasures of the palate, 138–41
　3. make your eating experience more enjoyable, 141–4
　4. don't settle, 144–5
　5. check in: does it still taste good?, 145–6
Polivy, Janet, 69–70, 82
Potter, John, 202
Primal food therapy, 70–1
Primal hunger, 63–4
Process thinking, 120–1
Professional Dieter, 9, 11–12, 13, 17
　eating style, 11
　problem, 11–12
Protein, as part of diet, 202–3
Pseudo-dieting, 45–7, 89–90
　becoming a vegetarian only for the purpose of losing weight, 47
　competing with someone else who is dieting, 46
　cutting back on food, 46
　eating at only certain times of the day, 45
　eating only "safe" foods, 45
　limiting carbohydrates, 46

meticulously counting fat grams, 45
pacifying hunger by drinking coffee or diet soda, 46
paying penance for eating "bad" foods, 46
putting on a "false food face" in public, 46
second-guessing or judging what you deserve to eat, 46–7
Psychological and emotional damage from dieting, 51
Punishment, using food as, 149, 151

Readiness to begin eating intuitively, 34–5
Rebel Ally, 98, 99, 106, 109, 110, 121
Rebound eating and weight gain, xv, 78–82, 213
　captivity behavior, 81
　Depression era eating, 81–2
　empty cupboard, the, 81
　food competition, 80
　once in a lifetime, 82
　one last shot, 82
Rebuilding positive food experiences, 37
Refuse-Not Unconscious Eater, 12–13, 16
Reject the diet mentality, principle, 20–1, 41–60
　diet void, the, 42–3
　Dieter's Dilemma, the, 47–8
　how to reject the diet mentality, 48–60
　Intuitive Eating tools, 60
　one-last-diet trap, the, 43–4
　pseudo-dieting, 45–7
Respect your body, principle, 27–8, 38, 39, 164–80
　body image, 166–7
　reaching your natural healthy weight, 176–9

Respect your body (*cont'd*)
saying good-bye to the fantasy,
179–80
why "respect," 167–76
"Restraint eating," 82–4
Restrained eating studies, 83–4
mind games—the
counterregulation effect, 83–4
perception affects eating, 84
Returning home syndrome, 80–1
Risk of premature death and heart
disease due to chronic dieting,
50, 68
Rodin, Judith, 166
Roth, Geneen, 211

Salivation increase with food
deprivation, 65
Satiety, comfortable, 125, 127, 132
Satisfaction from eating important,
136
avoid tension, 143
eat in a pleasant environment, 143
provide variety, 144
savor your food, 141–2
Satter, Ellyn, 15
Scales as false idols, 56–9
Scarsdale diet, 1
Sedation, using food as, 149, 150–1
Seesaw syndrome, the, 84–6
Seid, Roberta Pollack, 95
Self-awareness—the ultimate
weapon against the Food Police,
121–2
Self-fulfilling prophecies and
overeating, 90
Self-talk, 111–14
negative, and how to change it,
111, 113, 114–21
Self-trust and making peace with
food, 91–2
Sensory gratification, using food as,
149

Sensual qualities of food, 139–40
appearance, 140
aroma, 139
taste, 139
temperature, 140
texture, 139
volume or filling-capacity, 140
Serotonin, 66
Slim-Fast, 1, 3, 123
Smith, Anna Nicole, 165
Social influence and amount you eat,
131–2
Social withdrawal and dieting, 3
Soothing power of food, 153–4
Stacey, Michelle, 195
Starvation, study of, 61–3
Strength training, importance of,
190
Stress, coping with by eating, 154–5,
162–3
Suggested weights for adults, table
of, 178

Taste hunger, 75
*The 7 Habits of Highly Effective
People*, 48
TV diet food and diet product
commercials, 5–6

Unconditional permission to eat,
86–7
fears that hold you back, 88–92
five steps to making peace with
food, 92–3
peace process, the, 87–8
Unconscious Eater, 9, 12–13, 16
Chaotic, 9, 12, 16
Emotional, 13, 17
problem, 13
Refuse-Not, 12–13, 16
Waste-Not, 13, 16
University of Toronto study of
chronic dieters (1987), 95

U.S. Dietary Goals (1990), 177

Vegetarianism, 47

Waste-Not Unconscious Eater, 13, 16
Water, importance in the diet, 205
Weight-loss industry, xiii, 1, 9

Willpower, 62
  forget, 52–3
Wolf, Naomi, 63
Women's Health Trial (WHT), 209
Wooley, Susan, 51

Yo-yo dieting, 11, 50